GERD Diet Essentials

A Complete Food List for Flavorful, Heartburn-Free Living

Enhance Your Wellness with Delicious, Trigger-Free Recipes

Catherine Rosales-Holt, BSN, RN

Table of Contents

Chapter 1: Introduction

Welcome to GERD Diet Essentials: Your Roadmap to Heartburn-Free Living

Hey there! If you're holding this book, chances are you're intimately familiar with that unwelcome burning sensation in your chest, that sour taste that creeps up your throat, or the myriad of other uncomfortable symptoms that come with Gastroesophageal Reflux Disease, or GERD. You're not alone. Millions of people navigate the daily challenges of this condition, often feeling lost in a sea of conflicting information about what to eat and what to avoid.

That's precisely why this book, *GERD Diet Essentials*, was created – to be your trusted guide through the often-confusing world of GERD and nutrition. We're not about restrictive, joyless eating. Instead, we'll focus on empowering you with a comprehensive food list and delicious, trigger-free recipes that will help you take control of your symptoms and rediscover the pleasure of eating without the painful aftermath. Think of this as your practical toolkit for building a sustainable and flavorful diet that supports your well-being and helps you say goodbye to persistent heartburn.

Author's Journey: Catherine Rosales-Holt's Story – From Bedside to Your Bookshelf

My name is Catherine Rosales-Holt, and for over fifteen years, I've had the privilege of working as a registered nurse specializing in gastroenterology. Day in and day out, I've been alongside individuals just like you, listening to their struggles, answering their questions, and witnessing firsthand the profound impact that diet can have on managing GERD.

My journey into this specific area wasn't just professional; it became deeply personal. As a mother navigating the demands of family life, I understand the challenges of maintaining a healthy lifestyle amidst busy schedules and varying dietary needs. This personal understanding fuels my passion for helping others find practical and sustainable solutions for their health concerns.

Through my years of nursing, I've seen countless patients find significant relief and improved quality of life simply by making informed dietary choices. This experience solidified my belief that while medical treatments play a crucial role, nutrition is an equally powerful tool in managing GERD effectively. It's about more than just avoiding certain foods; it's about understanding *why* certain foods trigger symptoms and discovering a wide array of delicious alternatives that nourish your body without causing discomfort.

This book is born out of that experience – a desire to bridge the gap between medical knowledge and everyday living. I wanted to create a resource that is not only informative and evidence-based but also practical, approachable, and filled with recipes that you'll actually look forward to making.

How to Best Use This Guide: Your Companion on the Path to Digestive Comfort

Think of *GERD Diet Essentials* as your friendly companion on this journey. It's designed to be easy to navigate and packed with actionable information. Here's how you can get the most out of it:

- Familiarize Yourself with the Food Lists: The core of this book lies in the comprehensive food lists. Take the time to understand which foods are generally well-tolerated and which are common triggers. Remember that individual sensitivities can vary, so this guide provides a strong starting point for your own exploration.
- Explore the Recipes: Don't let dietary restrictions dampen your culinary spirit! The recipes included are specifically crafted to be GERD-friendly without sacrificing flavor. Experiment, adapt, and discover new favorite meals.
- Understand the "Why": We won't just tell you what to eat; we'll also touch upon the reasons behind certain dietary recommendations, empowering you to make informed choices even when you're not following a specific recipe.
- Use it as a Reference: Keep this book handy as you plan your meals, grocery shop, and even dine out. It's a quick and easy reference to help you make confident food decisions.
- Listen to Your Body: While this guide provides a solid foundation, remember that your body is unique. Pay attention to how different foods affect you and adjust your diet accordingly. This book is a starting point, and your personal experience is invaluable.

Why Catherine Rosales-Holt is an Authority on GERD and Nutrition: Bridging Medical Expertise with Real-Life Understanding

You might be wondering, "Why should I trust this author?" Here's why my background and experience make me a reliable guide on your GERD journey:

- Background in Nursing and Gastroenterology: My years as a registered nurse specializing in gastroenterology have provided me with a deep understanding of the digestive system and the intricacies of GERD. I've worked directly with patients, witnessed the impact of this condition, and stayed up-to-date on the latest medical advancements and treatment protocols.
- Experience in Dietary Management for GERD Patients: A significant part of my work involves educating patients on the crucial role of diet in managing their GERD symptoms. I've guided countless individuals through the process of identifying trigger foods, making sustainable dietary changes, and finding ways to enjoy eating again. This hands-on experience has given me invaluable insights into the practical challenges and successes of implementing a GERD-friendly diet.
- Commitment to Patient Education and Support: My passion lies in empowering individuals to take control of their health. I believe that clear, accessible information and ongoing support are essential for navigating chronic conditions like GERD. This book is an extension of that commitment – a resource designed to educate, encourage, and support you every step of the way.

Ultimately, my goal with *GERD Diet Essentials* is to empower you to live a life free from the constant discomfort of heartburn, without sacrificing delicious and satisfying meals. Let's embark on this journey together and discover the flavorful, heartburn-free life that awaits you.

Chapter 2: Understanding GERD: The Basics You Need to Know

Before we dive into the delicious world of GERD-friendly foods, let's take a moment to understand what Gastroesophageal Reflux Disease (GERD) actually is and why diet plays such a crucial role in managing it. Having a solid grasp of the fundamentals will empower you to make informed choices and truly understand how the food you eat can impact your symptoms.

What is Gastroesophageal Reflux Disease (GERD)? The Ups and Downs of Digestion

At its core, GERD is a digestive disorder that occurs when stomach acid or, occasionally, stomach contents flow back up into the esophagus. The esophagus is the tube that carries food from your mouth to your stomach. Normally, a muscular ring called the lower esophageal sphincter (LES) acts like a valve at the bottom of your esophagus. It relaxes to allow food and liquids to pass into your stomach and then tightens to prevent stomach contents from backing up.

In individuals with GERD, this LES either weakens or relaxes inappropriately, allowing stomach acid to reflux, or flow back, into the esophagus. This backflow can irritate the lining of the esophagus, leading to a variety of uncomfortable symptoms. Think of it like a one-way street where sometimes the traffic starts going in the wrong direction, causing congestion and irritation.

It's important to distinguish between occasional acid reflux, which many people experience from time to time, and GERD, which is a more chronic and often more severe condition. GERD is typically diagnosed when reflux occurs frequently (more than twice a week) or causes troublesome symptoms and/or complications.

Symptoms and Complications of GERD: More Than Just Heartburn

While heartburn – that burning sensation behind your breastbone – is the most common symptom of GERD, it's not the only one. The symptoms of GERD can vary from person to person and can range from mild to severe. Here are some of the common signs and symptoms:

- Heartburn: A burning pain in the chest that often occurs after eating and may be worse at night or when lying down.
- Regurgitation: The sensation of stomach contents, including sour liquid or food, backing up into your mouth or throat.
- Dysphagia: Difficulty swallowing or the feeling that food is stuck in your throat.
- Chronic Cough: Persistent coughing, especially at night, can be a symptom of stomach acid irritating the airways.
- Laryngitis or Hoarseness: Refluxed acid can irritate the vocal cords, leading to a sore throat, hoarseness, or a persistent need to clear your throat.
- Asthma-like Symptoms: In some cases, GERD can trigger or worsen asthma symptoms.

- Nausea and Vomiting: Although less common, some individuals with GERD may experience nausea or vomiting.
- Globus Sensation: The feeling of a lump in your throat, even when there's nothing there.
- Dental Erosion: Stomach acid can erode tooth enamel, leading to increased sensitivity and cavities.
- Sleep Disturbances: Nighttime reflux can disrupt sleep, leading to fatigue and reduced quality of life.

If left unmanaged, chronic GERD can lead to more serious complications, including:

- Esophagitis: Inflammation of the lining of the esophagus, which can cause pain, difficulty swallowing, and even bleeding.
- Esophageal Stricture: Narrowing of the esophagus due to scar tissue formation from chronic inflammation, making it difficult for food to pass.
- Barrett's Esophagus: A condition in which the lining of the esophagus changes to resemble the lining of the intestine. This is a precancerous condition and increases the risk of esophageal cancer.
- Esophageal Cancer: While relatively rare, chronic GERD is a significant risk factor for adenocarcinoma of the esophagus.

It's crucial to seek medical attention if you experience frequent or severe GERD symptoms to get a proper diagnosis and discuss appropriate management strategies.

The Importance of Diet in Managing GERD: You Are What You Eat (and What You Don't Eat)

Now, let's get to the heart of why this book is so important: the profound impact of diet on managing GERD. While medication and lifestyle changes play a role, the food you consume can significantly influence the frequency and severity of your reflux symptoms.

Think about it this way: the stomach acid that's causing the irritation is directly related to the digestive process, which is entirely dependent on what you eat and drink. Certain foods and beverages can:

- Increase Stomach Acid Production: Some items stimulate your stomach to produce more acid, increasing the likelihood of reflux.
- Relax the Lower Esophageal Sphincter (LES): Certain foods can cause the LES to relax, making it easier for stomach contents to flow back into the esophagus.
- Delay Gastric Emptying: When food stays in your stomach longer, there's a greater chance of reflux occurring.
- Directly Irritate the Esophageal Lining: Even mildly acidic foods can aggravate an already inflamed esophagus.

Conversely, a carefully chosen diet can help to:

- Reduce Stomach Acid Production: Opting for less acidic and less stimulating foods can help keep acid levels in check.
- Support Healthy LES Function: Avoiding foods that relax the LES can help it to function properly and prevent reflux.
- Promote Efficient Digestion: Choosing easily digestible foods can help your stomach empty at a normal rate, reducing the opportunity for reflux.

- Minimize Esophageal Irritation: Avoiding highly acidic or spicy foods can soothe an inflamed esophagus and prevent further irritation.

This is where the power of a GERD-friendly diet comes in. By understanding which foods are likely to trigger your symptoms and focusing on those that are well-tolerated, you can take significant steps towards managing your GERD and improving your overall well-being.

The following chapters will delve into specific food lists, providing you with clear guidance on what to enjoy and what to limit. We'll also explore delicious recipes that are designed to be both satisfying and gentle on your digestive system. Remember, managing GERD through diet isn't about deprivation; it's about making informed choices that nourish your body and help you live a more comfortable, heartburn-free life.

Chapter 3: The Basics of a GERD Diet: Your Foundation for Flavorful Relief

Now that we understand what GERD is and why diet matters, let's delve into the practicalities of a GERD diet. This chapter will lay the groundwork for making informed food choices and building a sustainable eating plan that helps minimize your symptoms and allows you to enjoy delicious meals.

What is a GERD Diet? It's More About Balance Than Restriction

A GERD diet isn't a rigid, one-size-fits-all prescription. Instead, it's a set of dietary guidelines focused on minimizing foods and eating habits that are known to trigger or worsen acid reflux. It's about finding a balance – identifying your personal trigger foods while embracing a wide variety of nourishing and flavorful options that are gentle on your digestive system.

Think of it as a personalized approach to eating that prioritizes foods that are less likely to:

- Stimulate excessive stomach acid production.
- Relax the lower esophageal sphincter (LES).
- Cause inflammation or irritation of the esophagus.
- Delay stomach emptying.

The goal isn't deprivation, but rather making smart swaps and incorporating cooking methods that support digestive health. It's about building a sustainable way of eating that allows you to manage your GERD symptoms effectively in the long term.

Key Principles of the GERD Diet: Your Guiding Stars

While individual triggers can vary, there are some core principles that form the foundation of a GERD-friendly diet:

1. Lowering Fat Intake: High-fat foods tend to slow down stomach emptying, which can increase the risk of reflux. They can also relax the LES. Opting for leaner proteins, low-fat dairy, and healthier fats in moderation is a key principle.
2. Reducing Acidity: Acidic foods and drinks can directly irritate the esophageal lining. Limiting citrus fruits, tomatoes and tomato-based products, vinegar, and acidic beverages can help reduce this irritation.
3. Avoiding Known Triggers: Certain foods and drinks are common GERD triggers for many people. These often include caffeine, alcohol, chocolate, peppermint and spearmint, and spicy foods. Identifying your personal triggers is crucial (more on this later).

4. Moderating Portion Sizes: Large meals can put pressure on the stomach and increase the likelihood of reflux. Eating smaller, more frequent meals throughout the day can be beneficial.

5. Eating Mindfully and Slowly: Rushing through meals can lead to swallowing more air and overeating, both of which can contribute to reflux.[10] Eating slowly and chewing thoroughly aids digestion.[11]

6. Staying Hydrated Wisely: While adequate hydration is important, the type and timing of your fluid intake can matter.[12] Water is generally the best choice. Avoid large amounts of fluids with meals, which can increase stomach volume.[13]

7. Timing Your Meals: Eating close to bedtime can increase the risk of nighttime reflux.[14] Aim to finish your last meal at least 2-3 hours before lying down.[15]

8. Gentle Cooking Methods: Opting for baking, broiling, grilling, steaming, or poaching over frying can significantly reduce the fat content of your meals.

Foods to Avoid and Foods to Embrace: Your Essential Grocery Guide

This is the information you've been waiting for! While individual sensitivities exist, these lists provide a general guideline for navigating the grocery store and your kitchen. Remember, this is a starting point, and you may find that you can tolerate some "avoid" foods in small amounts or prepared in specific ways. Keeping a food diary can be incredibly helpful in identifying your personal triggers.

Foods to Generally Avoid (Common GERD Triggers):

- High-Fat Foods: (e.g., fried foods, fatty meats, whole milk dairy, creamy sauces): Avoid because they slow stomach emptying and can relax the lower esophageal sphincter (LES), increasing reflux.
- Acidic Fruits and Vegetables: (e.g., citrus fruits and juices, tomatoes and tomato products): Avoid because their high acidity can directly irritate the inflamed lining of the esophagus.
- Spicy Foods: (e.g., chili peppers, hot sauces): Avoid as they can irritate the esophagus and potentially increase stomach acid production.
- Caffeine: (e.g., coffee, tea, soda, chocolate): Avoid because it can relax the LES, allowing stomach acid to back up.
- Alcohol: (e.g., beer, wine, spirits): Avoid as it can relax the LES and increase stomach acid production.
- Carbonated Beverages: (e.g., soda, sparkling water): Avoid because the bubbles can increase pressure in the stomach, leading to reflux.
- Mint: (e.g., peppermint, spearmint): Avoid as it can relax the LES, although some research shows this effect may be minimal at typical flavoring doses.
- Garlic and Onions (for some): Avoid if they are personal triggers, as they can sometimes increase stomach acid or cause digestive discomfort.
- Processed Foods: Avoid generally due to their often high fat, sodium, and additive content, which can irritate the digestive system.

Foods to Generally Embrace (GERD-Friendly Options):

- Lean Proteins: (e.g., chicken breast, fish, tofu, beans, lentils): Embrace as they are lower in fat and digest more easily, reducing the risk of prolonged stomach emptying and LES relaxation.
- Healthy Fats (in moderation): (e.g., avocado, olive oil, nuts, seeds): Embrace in moderation as they are less likely to trigger reflux than high amounts of unhealthy fats and are important for overall health.
- Non-Citrus Fruits: (e.g., bananas, melons, pears, apples, berries): Embrace as they are less acidic and gentler on the esophagus.
- Non-Acidic Vegetables: (e.g., leafy greens, broccoli, carrots, green beans, potatoes): Embrace as they are generally low in acid and well-tolerated.
- Whole Grains: (e.g., oatmeal, brown rice, quinoa, whole-wheat bread): Embrace as they are high in fiber, which promotes healthy digestion.
- Low-Fat Dairy (in moderation): (e.g., skim milk, low-fat yogurt, cottage cheese): Embrace in moderation as they are lower in fat and may be less likely to trigger reflux than full-fat options.
- Herbal Teas: (e.g., chamomile, ginger): Embrace as they are non-caffeinated and can sometimes have soothing properties for the digestive system.
- Water: Embrace as it's essential for hydration and doesn't contribute to stomach acid or LES relaxation.

Remember, this is a general guide. The next chapters will delve deeper into specific food lists and provide delicious recipes to help you put these principles into practice. The key is to listen to your body, experiment within these guidelines, and discover the GERD-friendly foods that work best for you.

Chapter 4: Decoding Food Labels – Your Secret Weapon Against GERD

I know that navigating food choices with GERD can feel like walking through a minefield sometimes. One minute you feel fine, the next, that familiar burn creeps up. While we know common triggers vary, the nutrition label on packaged foods can be an incredibly powerful tool to help you make informed choices and hopefully reduce those uncomfortable episodes.

Think of the nutrition facts panel and ingredients list as your personal detective kit. Let's break down what to look for:

1. Start with the Serving Size:

- Why it matters: Everything else on the label (calories, fat, sugar, etc.) is based on *one* serving. But be honest, how often do we *actually* eat just the listed serving size? Sometimes a small package contains 2 or 3 servings!
- GERD Connection: Eating large meals can put pressure on your stomach and the valve connecting it to your esophagus (the lower esophageal sphincter, or LES), potentially

causing reflux. Even if a food seems "safe" per serving, eating multiple servings at once can overload your system and increase fat or trigger ingredient intake.

- Your Action: Always check the "Serving Size" and "Servings Per Container" first. Then, be realistic about how much you plan to eat and adjust the other numbers accordingly. If you eat two servings, you need to double all the values!

2. Focus on Fat Content:

- Why it matters: High-fat foods are notorious GERD triggers for many people. Fat takes longer to digest, meaning food stays in your stomach longer, increasing the chance for reflux. Fat can also cause the LES to relax, making it easier for stomach contents to splash back up.
- Where to Look:
    - Total Fat: This gives you the overall picture. While some fat is necessary, aim for products lower in total fat, especially if fat is a known trigger for you. There's no single "magic number," but compare similar products and choose the lower-fat option when possible.
    - Saturated Fat & Trans Fat: These are generally less healthy fats, and foods high in them are often triggers (think fried foods, fatty meats, pastries, creamy sauces). Limiting these is good for both GERD and overall heart health.
- Your Action: Compare labels on similar items (e.g., different brands of crackers or yogurt). Choose options with lower Total Fat, Saturated Fat, and ideally 0g of Trans Fat. Be especially wary of items where fat contributes a large percentage of the total calories per serving.

3. Scan the Ingredients List – Your Trigger Checklist:

- Why it matters: This list tells you *what* is actually in the food, listed in descending order by weight. This is where you can spot specific ingredients known to aggravate GERD.
- Common Triggers to Watch For: *(I know I've already mentioned these but I need to put emphasis on this without having you flip the pages back and forth! 😁)*
    - Mint (Peppermint, Spearmint): Often found in gums, candies, teas, and sometimes desserts. Mint can relax the LES.
    - Chocolate/Cocoa: Another ingredient known to relax the LES.
    - Citrus Fruits/Acids (Citric Acid, Ascorbic Acid in high amounts): While necessary nutrients, high concentrations found in flavorings, juices, and preservatives can increase acidity. Look out for lemon, orange, lime, grapefruit flavorings or juices.
    - Tomato-Based Ingredients: Tomato paste, puree, sauce. Tomatoes are naturally acidic.
    - Onion & Garlic (often listed as powder or flavoring): Common triggers for many individuals.
    - Spicy Ingredients: Chili powder, cayenne, peppers, capsaicin, spices (sometimes listed vaguely – if you react to spice, be cautious).
    - Caffeine: May be listed outright or implied in ingredients like coffee, tea extracts, guarana.
    - (Sometimes) High Fructose Corn Syrup or Excessive Sugars: While not a direct trigger for everyone, very sugary items can sometimes accompany high-fat ingredients or simply contribute to overeating or weight gain, which can worsen GERD.

- Carbonation (listed as Carbonated Water): Found in sodas and sparkling water – the bubbles can increase stomach pressure.

- Your Action: Read the list carefully. If you know garlic bothers you, scan for "garlic powder." If you react to acidic foods, be wary of "citric acid" or tomato products, especially if they appear high up on the list (meaning there's more of it).

Putting It All Together: You're an Individual!

Remember, these are guidelines. Your personal triggers might be different. What causes severe heartburn for one person might be perfectly fine for you.

- ***Keep a Food Diary:*** This is invaluable. Note what you eat, *how much* you eat (link it back to serving sizes!), and any symptoms you experience. This helps you identify *your* specific patterns and triggers.
- ***Consider Cooking Methods:*** A food label tells you about the packaged product, but how you prepare it also matters. Frying adds fat, potentially making even a "safe" food problematic. Baking, grilling, or steaming are often better choices.
- ***Portion Size is Key:*** Even "safe" foods can cause reflux if eaten in very large quantities.

Reading labels takes a little practice, but it gets easier! By becoming familiar with serving sizes, fat content, and common trigger ingredients, you empower yourself to make choices that help you feel your best. Don't hesitate to bring labels or questions to your appointments with your doctor, or a registered dietitian – we're here to help you navigate your journey with GERD.

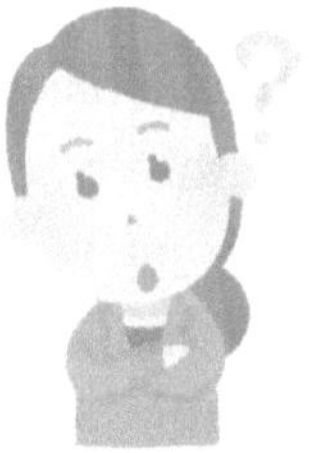

When looking at the labels, how much FAT should I look out for?

That's an excellent and very practical question! Patients often want a specific number to look for, and while I wish I could give you a single magic number, it's unfortunately not that simple when it comes to fat and GERD.

Thinking about the macronutrients, specifically fat:

1. **There's No Universal "Safe" Gram Amount:** The amount of fat that triggers GERD symptoms varies significantly from person to person. What one patient tolerates perfectly fine might cause immediate heartburn in another. Factors like your individual sensitivity, what else you're eating in that meal, and even your stress level that day can play a role.

2. **Focus on the *Overall Meal* Fat Content:** Instead of fixating on the grams of fat in *one* specific packaged item, it's more helpful to consider the total fat content of your entire meal. A small amount of fat from one source might be fine, but if you combine several moderate-fat items (e.g., avocado on toast with a side of sausage), the cumulative effect could trigger symptoms.

3. **Think "Lower" Rather Than a Specific Cut-Off:** When you're comparing similar products using the nutrition label:

    - *Compare and Choose*: Look at two brands of crackers, yogurts, or frozen meals side-by-side. Actively choose the one with the lower "Total Fat" per serving.

- *Be Wary of High Percentages:* Look at the % Daily Value (%DV) for Total Fat. While this is based on a general 2000-calorie diet, items with a very high %DV for fat (say, 20% or more *per serving*) are more likely to be problematic for GERD management, especially if you eat more than one serving or combine them with other fatty foods.
- *Check Fat's Calorie Contribution:* Fat has 9 calories per gram.[1] If a significant portion of a food's total calories comes from fat (you can estimate this: grams of fat * 9 = calories from fat), it's a higher-fat food. Be cautious with these.

4. **Prioritize *Avoiding Known High-Fat Categories*:** More important than a specific gram count on a label is recognizing and limiting foods that are generally high in fat. This includes:
   - Fried foods (French fries, fried chicken, doughnuts)
   - Creamy sauces and dressings (Alfredo sauce, ranch dressing, mayonnaise-heavy salads)
   - Fatty cuts of meat (ribeye steak, pork belly, sausage, bacon)
   - Full-fat dairy products (whole milk, heavy cream, rich cheeses, regular ice cream)
   - Pastries, pies, and rich desserts[2]
5. **Listen to Your Body & Use Your Food Diary:** This is truly the best way to determine *your* threshold. Note the food, the approximate portion size (relating it back to the label's serving size if possible), and any symptoms. You might find you can tolerate 10g of fat in one meal but not 15g, or that certain *types* of fatty foods are worse than others.

Instead of giving you a strict number like "avoid anything over X grams of fat," I advise you to:

- **Be a detective:** Use the label to compare products and consistently choose options lower in Total Fat and Saturated Fat.
- **Think about the whole plate:** Consider the total fat in the entire meal, not just one component.
- **Limit or avoid generally high-fat food categories** (fried, creamy, fatty meats, etc.).[3]
- **Pay close attention to portion sizes,** as more servings mean more fat.
- **Trust their own experience**: Use a food diary to learn their personal tolerance levels.

For truly personalized advice on macronutrient goals, including fat grams per day or per meal based on their total calorie needs and health status, I highly encourage you to consult with a Registered Dietitian. A dietitian can help you create a balanced plan that manages GERD while ensuring adequate nutrition.

Extensive List of Foods to Generally Embrace (GERD-Friendly Options)

I've compiled this more extensive list to provide you with a wider variety of delicious and gentle options to incorporate into your diet. Remember, individual tolerances can vary, so pay attention to how your body responds to different foods.

LEAN PROTEINS

(Lower in fat, digest easily, reduce prolonged stomach emptying and LES relaxation)

- POULTRY (Skinless)
  - Chicken breast (baked, grilled, poached, or steamed)
  - Turkey breast (baked, grilled, poached, or steamed)
  - Lean ground chicken or turkey
- FISH:
  - White fish (cod, haddock, flounder, tilapia, snapper - baked, grilled, poached, or steamed)
  - Fatty fish (salmon, tuna, mackerel, sardines - baked, grilled, or poached, consume in moderation due to fat content, but rich in omega-3s)

PLANT-BASED PROTEINS

- Tofu (firm or extra-firm, prepared in GERD-friendly ways like baking, stir-frying with minimal oil)
- Tempeh (steamed, baked, or lightly stir-fried)
- Beans (black beans, kidney beans, cannellini beans, navy beans - well-cooked and in moderation to minimize gas)
- Lentils (all types - well-cooked and in moderation)
- Edamame (steamed or shelled)
- Peas (green peas, split peas)
- Quinoa (a complete protein)

HEALTHY FATS

(in Moderation): (Less likely to trigger reflux than high amounts of unhealthy fats, important for overall health)

- Avocado: Enjoy in moderation; can be creamy and satisfying.
- Olive Oil: Use for cooking and dressings in moderation. Extra virgin olive oil is a good choice.
- Nuts (Unsalted, Plain):
- Almonds
- Walnuts
- Pecans
- Cashews
- Pistachios
- Chia seeds
- Flax seeds (ground)
- Pumpkin seeds (pepitas)
- Sunflower seeds
- Nut Butters (Natural, No Added Sugar or Oils): Almond butter, peanut butter (in moderation), cashew butter.

NON-CITRUS FRUITS:

(Less acidic and gentler on the esophagus)

- Melons:
    - Cantaloupe
    - Honeydew melon
    - Watermelon
- Bananas: Ripe bananas are generally well-tolerated.
- Pears: Choose ripe pears.
- Apples: Sweet varieties like Gala, Fuji, or Honeycrisp (peeled may be better for some).
- Dates: In moderation.
- Berries:
    - Blueberries
    - Strawberries (in moderation, some individuals may find them slightly acidic)
    - Raspberries (in moderation)
    - Blackberries (in moderation)
- Peaches: Ripe peaches.
- Mangoes: Ripe mangoes.
- Papaya

NON-ACIDIC VEGETABLES: (GENERALLY LOW IN ACID AND WELL-TOLERATED)

- Leafy Greens:
  - Lettuce (romaine, butter, green leaf)
  - Spinach
  - Kale (cooked)
  - Swiss chard (cooked)
- Cruciferous Vegetables (well-cooked):
  - Broccoli
  - Cauliflower
  - Cabbage (in moderation, may cause gas for some)
- Brussels sprouts (in moderation, may cause gas for some)
- Root Vegetables:
  - Carrots
  - Potatoes (baked, boiled, mashed with low-fat milk)
  - Sweet potatoes (baked, boiled, mashed)
  - Beets
  - Turnips
- Squash:
  - Zucchini
  - Yellow squash
  - Butternut squash
  - Acorn squash
- Green Vegetables:
  - Green beans
  - Peas
  - Asparagus
- Other Vegetables:
  - Cucumbers
  - Mushrooms
  - Onions (cooked in small amounts, can be a trigger for some raw)
  - Garlic (cooked in small amounts, can be a trigger for some raw)
  - Celery

WHOLE GRAINS: (HIGH IN FIBER, PROMOTE HEALTHY DIGESTION)

- Oatmeal: Plain, unsweetened.
- Brown Rice
- Quinoa
- Whole-Wheat Bread: Look for varieties with minimal additives.
- Whole-Grain Pasta
- Barley
- Farro
- Spelt

LOW-FAT DAIRY (IN MODERATION):

(Lower in fat, may be less likely to trigger reflux than full-fat options)

- Skim Milk:
- Low-Fat (1% or 2%) Milk:
- Low-Fat Yogurt: Plain, unsweetened Greek or regular yogurt.
- Low-Fat Cottage Cheese

HERBAL TEAS: (NON-CAFFEINATED, CAN HAVE SOOTHING PROPERTIES)

- Herbal Teas: (Non-caffeinated, can have soothing properties)
- Chamomile Tea: Known for its calming effects.
- Ginger Tea: May help with nausea and digestion.
- Licorice Root Tea (DGL form): Deglycyrrhizinated licorice (DGL) may have soothing properties for the esophagus, but consult your doctor before regular use.
- Fennel Tea: May help with bloating and digestion.
- Marshmallow Root Tea: May have a soothing effect on the digestive tract.
- Slippery Elm Tea: May coat and soothe the esophagus.

General Food List Reference

As I have mentioned earlier in this chapter, the point in managing GERD is not being able to religiously follow a standardized magic number of specific nutrients in your diet but to avoid unmistakable triggers and be able to gauge your tolerance level of some foods.

The key is in moderation.

The following section on this chapter is a general food list guide which is not only beneficial for patients suffering from GERD but can virtually be used by anybody to check out their own nutrient consumption. This will come really handy after you visit your Dietitian who will give you more insights on your individual, specific macro and micronutrient consumption daily.

How to use the charts

Refer to the charts to check for the macronutrient and micronutrient values according to the general standard recommendations I have mentioned or as set by your dietitian.

1. The foods are categorized: Vegetables, vegetable proteins, Fruits, Carbohydrates, Milks and Cheeses, Fats and Oils, Animal Proteins, and Herbs & Spices.

2. Each food item is given at least 1 corresponding serving size. We have standardized the serving size to 100 grams, but you will also find other alternative serving sizes to most food items in the charts.

    a. For reference:

G/g = grams	c = cup
mg = milligrams	tsp = teaspoon
svg = serving	tbsp = tablespoon
fl oz = fluid ounce	pc = piece

3. How to read/apply the chart?

For example, you are only allowed to have around 140mg of Potassium for your snack, and you have 1 peach on hand. Looking at the chart, 1 piece medium-sized raw peach is 150grams, with 285 mg of Potassium. If you have a scale handy, you may want to weigh 75grams only of the peach you have. Or you can just simply slice the peach into half and just eat half of it.

PEACHES	SERVING QUANTITY	SERVING UNIT	CALORIES (kcal)	PROTEIN (g)	TOTAL CARBOHYDRATES (g)	SODIUM (mg)	POTASSIUM (mg)	PHOSPHORUS (mg)	TOTAL FAT (g)
raw, medium	100.00	g	39	0.9	9.5	0.00	190.0	20.00	0.25
approx.	150.00	g	59	1.4	14.3	0.00	285.0	30.00	0.38
	1.00	pc/ item							

A. Vegetables

Hey there!

Do you need to print out this Food List?

You can download a printable version of this chart by scanning the QR code below or copying the link on your computer browser.

https://go.renaltracker.com/printfoodlist

ASPARAGUS	SERVING QUANTITY	SERVING UNIT	CALORIES (kCal)	PROTEIN (g)	TOTAL CARBOHYDRATES (g)	SODIUM (mg)	POTASSIUM (mg)	PHOSPHORUS (mg)	TOTAL FAT (g)
boiled, drained	100.00	g	22	2.4	4.1	14.00	224.0	54.00	0.22
	90.00	g	20	2.2	3.7	12.60	201.6	48.60	0.20
	0.50	c							
frozen	100.00	g	24	3.2	4.1	8.00	253.0	64.00	0.23
	87.00	g	21	2.8	3.6	6.96	220.1	55.68	0.20
	6.00	pcs							
frozen, boiled, drained	100.00	g	18	3.0	1.9	3.00	172.0	49.00	0.42
	90.00	g	16	2.7	1.7	2.70	154.8	44.10	0.38
	0.50	c							
canned, drained	100.00	g	19	2.1	2.5	287.0	172.0	43.00	0.65
	121.00	g	23	2.6	3.0	347.2	208.1	52.03	0.79
	0.50	c							
BEANS									
green wax, raw	100.00	g	31	1.8	7.0	6.00	211.0	38.00	
	82.50	g	26	1.5	5.8	4.95	174.1	31.35	
	0.75	c							
green wax, frozen	100.00	g	33	1.8	7.5	3.00	186.0	32.00	
	82.67	g	27	1.5	6.2	2.48	153.7	26.45	
	0.67	c							
green wax, boiled, drained	100.00	g	35	1.9	7.9	1.00	146.0	29.00	
	125.00	g	44	2.4	9.9	1.25	182.5	36.25	
	1.00	c							
green wax, canned, drained	100.00	g	21	1.1	4.2	268.0	96.00	22.00	
	135.00	g	28	1.4	5.7	361.8	129.6	29.70	
	1.00	c							
CARROTS									
strips, slices	100.00	g	41	0.9	9.6	69.00	320.0	35.00	
	122.00	g	50	1.1	11.7	84.18	390.4	42.70	
	1.00	c							
grated	100.00	g	41	0.9	9.6	69.00	320.0	35.00	
	82.50	g	34	0.8	7.9	56.93	264.0	28.88	
	0.75	c							
sliced,boiled drained, no salt	100.00	g	35	0.8	8.2	58.00	235.0	30.00	
	78.00	g	27	0.6	6.4	45.24	183.3	23.40	
	0.50	c							
frozen	100.00	g	36	0.8	7.9	68.00	235.0	33.00	
	85.33	g	31	0.7	6.7	58.03	200.5	28.16	
	0.67	c							
baby	100.00	g	35	0.6	8.2	78.00	237.0	28.00	
	80.00	g	28	0.5	6.6	62.40	189.6	22.40	
	8.00	pcs							
juice, canned	100.00	g	40	1.0	9.3	66.00	292.0	42.00	
	236.00	g	94	2.2	21.9	155.7	689.1	99.12	
	8.00	fl oz							

TOMATO

TOMATO	SERVING QUANTITY	SERVING UNIT	CALORIES (KCal)	PROTEIN (g)	TOTAL CARBOHYDRATES (g)	SODIUM (mg)	POTASSIUM (mg)	PHOSPHORUS (mg)	TOTAL FAT (g)
red, whole	100.00	g	18	0.9	3.9	5.00	237	24.00	
medium 2.6 in	123.00	g	22	1.1	4.8	6.15	292	29.52	
diameter	1.00	pc							
diced or	100.00	g	18	0.9	3.9	5.00	237	24.00	
chopped	90.00	g	16	0.8	3.5	4.50	213	21.60	
	0.50	c							
yellow,	100.00	g	15	1.0	3.0	23.00	258	36.00	
chopped	92.67	g	14	0.9	2.8	21.31	239	33.36	
	0.67	c							
orange,	100.00	g	16	1.2	3.2	42.00	212	29.00	
chopped	79.00	g	13	0.9	2.5	33.18	167	22.91	
	0.50	c							
green	100.00	g	23	1.2	5.1	13.00	204	28.00	
	90.00	g	21	1.1	4.6	11.70	183	25.20	
	0.50	c							
whole, canned	100.00	g	16	0.8	3.5	115	191	17.00	
	240.00	g	38	1.9	8.3	276	458	40.80	
	1.00	c							
sauce, canned,	100.00	g	24	1.2	5.3	11.00	297	27.00	
no salt	244.00	g	59	2.9	13.0	26.84	725	65.88	
	1.00	c							
crushed,	100.00	g	32	1.6	7.3	186	293	32.00	
canned	56.70	g	18	0.9	4.1	106	166	18.14	
	2.00	oz							
paste, canned	100.00	g	82	4.3	18.9	790	1,014	83.00	
	32.80	g	27	1.4	6.2	259	333	27.22	
	2.00	tbsp							
puree, canned,	100.00	g	38	1.7	9.0	28.00	439	40.00	
no salt	250.00	g	95	4.1	22.5	70.00	1,098	100.00	
	1.00	c							
sun dried, in	100.00	g	213	5.1	23.3	266	1,565	139.00	
oil, drained	27.50	g	59	1.4	6.4	73.15	430	38.23	
	0.25	c							
Ketchup, low	100.00	g	101	1.0	27.4	20.00	281	26.00	
sodium	15.00	g	15	0.2	4.1	3.00	42.15	3.90	
	1.00	tbsp							
juice, canned	100.00	g	17	0.9	3.5	253	217	19.00	
	243.00	g	41	2.1	8.6	614	527	46.17	
	8.00	fl oz							
cherry, sweet,	100.00	g	63	1.1	16.0	0.00	222	21.00	
raw	138.00	g	87	1.5	22.1	0.00	306	29.00	
	1.00	c							

PEPPER

PEPPER	SERVING QUANTITY	SERVING UNIT	CALORIES (kCal)	PROTEIN (g)	TOTAL CARBOHYDRATES (g)	SODIUM (mg)	POTASSIUM (mg)	PHOSPHORUS (mg)	TOTAL FAT (g)
bell, sweet yellow, 3 in diameter	100.00	g	27	1.0	6.3	2.00	212.0	24.00	
	186.00	g	50	1.9	11.8	3.72	394.3	44.64	
	1.00	pc							
bell, sweet green, chopped	100.00	g	20	0.9	4.6	3.00	175.0	20.00	
	74.50	g	15	0.6	3.5	2.24	130.3	14.90	
	0.50	c							
bell, sweet green, sauteed	100.00	g	116	0.8	4.2	17.00	134.0	15.00	
bell, sweet red, chopped	100.00	g	26	1.0	6.0	4.00	211.0	26.00	
	74.50	g	19	0.7	4.5	2.98	157.2	19.37	
	0.50	c							
bell, sweet red, sauteed	100.00	g	133	1.0	6.6	21.00	193.0	23.00	
bell, sweet red, chopped, frozen, drained, boiled, no salt added	100.00	g	16	1.0	3.3	4.00	72.00	13.00	
	85.05	g	14	0.8	2.8	3.40	61.24	11.06	
	3.00	oz							
jalapeno, sliced	100.00	g	29	0.9	6.5	3.00	248.0	26.00	
	22.50	g	7	0.2	1.5	0.68	55.80	5.85	
	0.13	c							
serrano, chopped	100.00	g	32	1.7	6.7	10.00	305.0	40.00	
	26.25	g	8	0.5	1.8	2.63	80.06	10.50	
	0.25	c							
black, ground	100.00	g	251	10.4	64.0	20.00	1,329	158.0	
	2.10	g	5	0.2	1.3	0.42	27.91	3.32	
	1.00	tsp							
white, ground	100.00	g	296	10.4	68.6	5.00	73.00	176.0	
	2.40	g	7	0.3	1.7	0.12	1.75	4.22	
	1.00	tsp							
Hot chilli, red	100.00	g	40	1.9	8.8	9.00	322.0	43.00	
	45.00	g	18	0.8	4.0	4.05	144.9	19.35	
	1.00	pc							

CABBAGE	SERVING QUANTITY	SERVING UNIT	CALORIES (KCal)	PROTEIN (g)	TOTAL CARBOHYDRATES (g)	SODIUM (mg)	POTASSIUM (mg)	PHOSPHORUS (mg)	TOTAL FAT (g)
green, chopped	100.00	g	25	1.3	5.8	18.00	170.0	26.00	
	89.00	g	22	1.1	5.2	16.02	151.3	23.14	
	1.00	c							
green shredded, sliced	100.00	g	25	1.3	5.8	18.00	170.0	26.00	
	87.50	g	22	1.1	5.1	15.75	148.7	22.75	
	1.25	c							
green, shredded, boiled, drained, no salt added	100.00	g	23	1.3	5.5	8.00	196.0	33.00	
	75.00	g	17	1.0	4.1	6.00	147.0	24.75	
	0.50	c							
chinese, shredded, raw	100.00	g							
	76.00	g	12	0.9		6.84	181.0	22.04	
	1.00	c							
chinese, cooked, no salt	100.00	g							
	75.00	g	17	1.0		6.00	147.0	24.75	
	0.50	c							
red, shredded	100.00	g	31	1.4	7.4	27.00	243.0	30.00	
	87.50	g	27	1.3	6.5	23.63	212.6	26.25	
	1.25	c							
red, shredded, boiled, drained, no salt added	100.00	g	29	1.5	6.9	28.00	262.0	33.00	
	75.00	g	27	1.1	5.2	21.00	196.5	24.75	
	0.50	c							
Bok Choy or White Mustard, shredded	100.00	g	13	1.5	2.2	65.00	252.0	37.00	
	87.50	g	11	1.3	1.9	56.88	220.5	32.38	
	1.25	c							
Bok Choy/ Pak Choi,shredded, boiled, drained	100.00	g	12	1.6	1.8	34.00	371.0	29.00	
	85.00	g	10	1.3	1.5	28.90	315.3	24.65	
	0.50	c							
Kimchi	100.00	g	15	1.1	2.4	498.0	151.0	24.00	
	150.00	g	23	1.7	3.6	747.0	226.5	36.00	
	1.00	c							

MUSHROOM	SERVING QUANTITY	SERVING UNIT	CALORIES (KCal)	PROTEIN (g)	TOTAL CARBOHYDRATES (g)	SODIUM (mg)	POTASSIUM (mg)	PHOSPHORUS (mg)	TOTAL FAT (g)
Shitake, raw	100.00	g	34	2.2	6.8	9.00	304	112.0	
	19.00	g	6	0.4	1.3	1.71	57.76	21.28	
	1.00	pc							
Shitake, dried	100.00	g	296	9.6	75.4	13.00	1,534	294.0	
	32.40	g	96	3.1	24.4	4.21	497	95.26	
	9.00	pcs							
Shitake, cooked	100.00	g	56	1.6	14.4	4.00	117	29.00	
	72.50	g	41	1.1	10.4	2.90	84.83	21.03	
	0.50	c							
Shitake, stir fried	100.00	g	39	3.5	7.7	5.00	326	111.0	
	108.00	g	42	3.7	8.3	5.40	352	119.9	
	1.00	c							
Portabella/ Portabello	100.00	9	22	2.1	3.9	9.00	364	108.0	
Portabello, grilled	100.00	g	29	3.3	4.4	11.00	437	135.0	
White, raw	100.00	g	22	3.0	3.3	5.00	318	86.00	
	96.00	g	21	3.0	3.1	4.80	305	82.56	
	1.00	c							
white, sliced, stir-fried	100.00	g	26	3.6	4.0	12.00	396	105.0	
	108.00	g	28	3.9	4.4	12.96	428	113.4	
	1.00	c							
LETTUCE									
romaine, shredded	100.00	g	17	1.2	3.3	8.00	247.0	30.00	
	70.50	g	12	0.9	2.3	5.64	174.1	21.15	
	1.50	c							
butterhead, medium leaves	100.00	g	13	1.4	2.2	5.00	238.0	33.00	
	82.50	g	11	1.1	1.8	4.13	196.3	27.23	
	11.00	pcs							
Red Leaf, shredded	100.00	g	13	1.3	2.3	25	187	28.00	
	28.00	g	4	0.4	0.6	7	52.36	7.84	
	1.00	c							
Iceberg, shredded or chopped	100.00	g	14	0.9	3.0	10	141	20.00	
	108.00	g	15	1.0	3.2	11	152.3	21.60	
	1.50	c							
Iceberg, loose leaves, medium	100.00	g	14	0.9	3.0	10	141.0	20.00	
	80.00	g	11	0.7	2.4	8	112.8	16.00	
	10.00	pcs							

CORN

	SERVING QUANTITY	SERVING UNIT	CALORIES (KCal)	PROTEIN (g)	TOTAL CARBOHYDRATES (g)	SODIUM (mg)	POTASSIUM (mg)	PHOSPHORUS (mg)	TOTAL FAT (g)
white, sweet	100.00	g	390	7.8	86.6	956.0	88.00	39.00	
	25.00	g	98	2.0	21.7	239.0	22.00	9.75	
	1.00	c							
white, steamed (Navajo)	100.00	g	386	9.7	75.2	4.00	532.0	312.0	
	85.05	g	328	8.3	64.0	3.40	452.4	265.3	
	3.00	oz							
white, stew, steamed (Navajo)	100.00	g	112	8.8	10.8	104.0	177.0	107.0	
	85.05	g	95	7.5	9.2	88.45	150.5	91.00	
	3.00	oz							
sweet, boiled, drained	100.00	g	94	3.1	22.3	4.00	251.0	75.00	0.74
	82.00	g	77	2.6	18.3	3.28	205.8	61.50	0.61
	0.50	c							
flour, white, whole grain	100.00	g	361	6.9	76.9	5.00	315.0	272.0	3.86
	29.25	g	106	2.0	22.5	1.46	92.14	79.56	1.13
	0.25	c							
yellow, sweet, boiled, drained	100.00	g	96	3.4	21.0	1.00	218.0	77.00	1.50
	82.00	g	79	2.8	17.2	0.82	178.7	63.14	1.23
	0.50	c							
yellow, sweet, on the cob	100.00	g	86	3.3	18.7	15.00	270.0	89.00	1.35
	154.00	g	77	2.9	16.8	13.50	243.0	80.10	1.22
	1.00	c							
yellow, sweet, creamed, canned	100.00	g	72	1.7	18.1	261.0	134.0	51.00	0.42
	128.00	g	92	2.2	23.2	334.0	171.5	65.28	0.54
	0.50	c							
yellow, sweet, kernels, frozen	100.00	g	88	3.0	20.7	3.00	213.0	70.00	0.78
	82.00	g	72	2.5	17.0	2.46	174.6	57.40	0.64
	0.50	c							
yellow, sweet, canned with liquid	100.00	g	61	2.0	13.9	195.0	136.0	46.00	0.77
	128.00	g	78	2.5	17.7	249.6	174.0	58.88	0.99
	0.50	c							
tortilla, no salt added	100.00	g	222	5.7	46.6	11.00	154.0	314.0	2.50
	26.00	g	58	1.5	12.1	2.86	40.04	81.64	0.65
	1.00	pc							

	SERVING QUANTITY	SERVING UNIT	CALORIES (kCal)	PROTEIN (g)	TOTAL CARBOHYDRATES (g)	SODIUM (mg)	POTASSIUM (mg)	PHOSPHORUS (mg)	TOTAL FAT (g)
BROCCOLI									
florets, raw	100.00	g	28	3.0	5.1	27.00	325.0	66.00	0.35
	71.00	g	20	2.1	3.6	19.17	230.7	46.86	0.25
	1.00	c							
Cooked, no salt	100.00	g	35	2.4	7.2	41.00	293.0	67.00	0.41
	78.00	g	27	1.9	5.6	31.98	228.5	52.26	0.32
	0.50	c							
frozen, spears	100.00	g	29	3.1	5.4	17.00	250.0	59.00	0.34
	85.05	g	25	2.6	4.6	14.46	212.6	50.18	0.29
	3.00	oz							
CAULIFLOWER									
green, raw	100.00	g	31	3.0	6.1	23.00	300.0	62.00	0.30
	64.00	g	20	1.9	3.9	14.72	192.0	39.68	0.19
	1.00	c							
cooked, no salt	100.00	g	32	3.0	6.3	23.00	278.0	57.00	0.31
	62.00	g	20	1.9	3.9	14.26	172.3	35.34	0.19
	0.50	c							
CUCUMBER									
sliced, raw	100.00	g	15	0.7	3.6	2.00	147.0	24.00	0.11
	52.00	g	8	0.3	1.9	1.04	76.44	12.48	0.06
	0.50	c							
sliced	100.00	g	15	0.7	3.6	2.00	147.0	24.00	0.11
	78.00	g	12	0.5	2.8	1.56	114.6	18.72	0.09
	0.75	c							
BEETS									
raw	100.00	g	43	1.6	9.6	78.00	325.0	40.00	0.17
	90.67	g	39	1.5	8.7	70.72	294.6	36.27	0.15
	0.67	c							
whole or sliced, boiled, drained, no salt	100.00	g	44	1.7	10.0	77.00	305.0	38.00	0.18
Whole, canned	100.00	g	30	0.7	7.1	143.00	159.0	15.00	0.09
	246.00	g	74	1.8	17.6	351.78	391.1	36.90	0.22
	1.00	c							
sliced, canned, drained	100.00	g	31	0.9	7.2	194.00	148.0	17.00	0.14
	85.00	g	26	0.8	6.1	164.90	125.8	14.45	0.12
	0.50	c							

PEAS

PEAS	SERVING QUANTITY	SERVING UNIT	CALORIES (kCal)	PROTEIN (g)	TOTAL CARBOHYDRATES (g)	SODIUM (mg)	POTASSIUM (mg)	PHOSPHORUS (mg)	TOTAL FAT (g)
green	100.00	g	81	5.4	14.5	5.00	244.0	108.0	0.40
	72.50	g	59	3.9	10.5	3.63	176.9	78.30	0.29
	0.50	c							
green, frozen	100.00	g	77	5.2	13.6	108.0	153.0	82.00	0.40
	72.00	g	55	3.8	9.8	77.76	110.1	59.04	0.29
	0.50	c							
green, boiled, drained	100.00	g	84	5.4	15.6	3.00	271.0	117.0	0.22
	80.00	g	67	4.3	12.5	2.40	216.8	93.60	0.18
	0.50	c							
green, canned, drained	100.00	g	68	4.5	11.4	273.0	106.0	67.00	0.80
	87.50	g	60	3.9	9.9	238.8	92.7	58.63	0.70
	0.50	c							
green, frozen, boiled, drained	100.00	g	78	5.2	14.3	72.00	110.0	77.00	0.27
	80.00	g	62	4.1	11.4	57.60	88.00	61.60	0.22
	0.50	c							
split, boiled, no salt added	100.00	g	118	8.3	21.1	2.00	362.0	99.00	0.39
	98.00	g	116	8.2	21.0	1.96	354.7	97.02	0.38
	0.50	c							
sugar or snow peas, whole fresh	100.00	g	42	2.8	7.6	4.00	200.0	53.00	0.20
	78.75	g	33	2.2	6.0	3.15	157.5	41.74	0.16
	1.25	c							
snow/sugar, frozen	100.00	g	42	2.8	7.6	4.00	200.0	53.00	0.20
	78.75	g	33	2.2	6.0	3.15	157.5	41.74	0.16
	1.25	c							
snow/sugar, boiled, drained	100.00	g	42	3.3	7.1	4.00	240.0	55.00	0.23
	80.00	g	34	2.6	5.6	3.20	192.0	44.00	0.18
	0.50	c							
snow/sugar, frozen, boiled, drained	100.00	g	52	3.5	9.0	5.00	217.0	58.00	0.38
	80.00	g	42	2.8	7.2	4.00	173.6	46.40	0.30
	0.50	c							

POTATOES	SERVING QUANTITY	SERVING UNIT	CALORIES (kCal)	PROTEIN (g)	TOTAL CARBOHYDRATES (g)	SODIUM (mg)	POTASSIUM (mg)	PHOSPHORUS (mg)	TOTAL FAT (g)
russet, flesh and skin	100.00	g	79	2.1	18.1	5.00	417.0	55.00	0.08
russet, flesh and skin, baked	100.00	g	95	2.6	21.4	14.00	550.0	71.00	0.13
	173.00	g	164	4.6	37.1	24.22	951.5	122.8	0.22
	1.00	pc							
white, flesh and skin	100.00	g	69	1.7	15.7	16.00	407.0	62.00	0.10
white, flesh and skin, baked	100.00	g	92	2.1	21.1	7.00	544.0	75.00	0.15
	173.00	g	159	3.6	36.5	12.11	941.1	129.7	0.26
	1.00	pcs							
French fries, frozen	100.00	g	147	2.2	24.8	332.0	408.0	83.00	4.66
	71.50	g	105	1.6	17.7	237.3	291.7	59.35	3.33
	11.00	pcs							
sweet, cubed	100.00	g	86	1.6	20.1	55.00	337.0	47.00	0.05
	99.75	g	86	1.6	20.1	54.86	336.1	46.88	0.05
	0.75	c							
sweet, boiled, mashed	100.00	g	76	1.4	17.7	27.00	230.0	32.00	0.14
	328.00	g	249	4.5	58.1	88.56	754.4	105	0.46
	1.00	c							
sweet, frozen, baked	100.00	g	100	1.7	23.4	8.00	377.0	44.00	0.12
	117.33	g	117	2.0	27.5	9.39	442.3	51.63	0.14
	0.67	c							
sweet, baked, peeled	100.00	g	90	2.0	20.7	36.00	475.0	54.00	0.15
	0.50	c							
chips, unsalted	100.00	g	536	7.0	52.9	8.00	1,275	165.0	34.60
	28.35	g	152	2.0	15.0	2.27	361.4	46.78	9.81
	1.00	oz							
hash browns, frozen	100.00	g	82	2.1	17.7	22.00	285.0	47.00	0.62
	70.00	g	57	1.4	12.4	15.40	199.5	32.90	0.43
	0.33	c							
wedges, frozen	100.00	g	129	2.7	25.5	49.00	394.0	87.00	2.20

ARTI-CHOKES	SERVING QUANTITY	SERVING UNIT	CALORIES (kCal)	PROTEIN (g)	TOTAL CARBOHYDRATES (g)	SODIUM (mg)	POTASSIUM (mg)	PHOSPHORUS (mg)	TOTAL FAT (g)
whole, boiled, drained	100.00	g	53	2.9	12.0	60.00	286	73.00	0.34
med size	120.00	g	64	3.5	14.3	72.00	343	87.60	0.41
	1.00	pc							
hearts, boiled, drained	100.00	g	53	2.9	11.9	60.00	286	73.00	0.34
	84.00	g	45	2.4	10.0	50.40	240	61.32	0.29
	0.50	c							
Globe or French, frozen	100.00	g	45	3.1	9.2	53.00	264	61.00	0.50
boiled, drained	80.00	g	36	2.5	7.3	42.40	211	48.80	0.40
1 svg= 1/3 of 9oz package	1.00	svg							
ALFALFA									
sprouts	100.00	g	23	4.0	2.1	6.00	79.00	70.00	0.69
	33.00	g	8	1.3	0.7	1.98	26.07	23.10	0.23
	1.00	c							
CELERY									
stalk	100.00	g	14	0.7	3.0	80.00	260	24.00	0.17
medium 7.5 - 8 in long	80.00	g	11	0.6	2.4	64.00	208	19.20	0.14
	2.00	stalks							
diced, chopped	100.00	g	14	0.7	3.0	80.00	260	24.00	0.17
	101.00	g	14	0.7	3.0	80.80	263	24.24	0.17
	1.00	c							
celeriac or celery root	100.00	g	42	1.5	9.2	100.0	300	115	0.30
	78.00	g	33	1.2	7.2	78.00	234	90	0.23
	0.50	c							
seeds	100.00	g	392	18.1	41.4	160.0	1,400	547	25.27
	2.00	g	8	0.4	0.8	3.20	28.00	10.94	0.51
	1.00	tsp							
flakes, dried	100.00	g	319	11.3	68.7	1,435	4,388	402	2.10
	28.35	g	90	3.2	18.1	406.8	1,244	114	0.60
	1.00	oz							

COLLARDS	SERVING QUANTITY	SERVING UNIT	CALORIES (kCal)	PROTEIN (g)	TOTAL CARBOHYDRATES (g)	SODIUM (mg)	POTASSIUM (mg)	PHOSPHORUS (mg)	TOTAL FAT (g)
chopped, raw	100.00	g	32	3.0	5.4	17.00	213.0	25.00	0.61
	90.00	g	29	2.7	4.9	15.30	191.7	22.50	0.55
	2.50	c							
boiled, drained	100.00	g	33	2.7	5.7	15.00	117.0	32.00	0.72
	95.00	g	31	2.6	5.4	14.25	111.1	30.40	0.68
	0.50	c							
frozen, chopped, raw	100.00	g	33	2.7	6.5	48.00	253.0	27.00	0.37
	85.05	g	28	2.3	5.5	40.82	215.1	22.96	0.31
	3.00	oz							
frozen, chopped, boiled/ drained	100.00	g	36	3.0	7.1	50.00	251.0	27.00	0.41
	85.00	g	31	2.5	6.0	42.50	213.3	22.95	0.35
	0.50	c							
EGGPLANT/AUBERGINE									
boiled, drained, no salt cut in 1" cubes	100.00	g	35	0.8	8.7	1.00	123.0	15.00	0.23
	99.00	g	35	0.8	8.6	0.99	121.7	14.85	0.23
	1.00	c							
pickled	100.00	g	49	0.9	9.8	1,674	12.00	9.00	0.70
	136	g	67	1.2	13.3	2,276	16.32	12.24	0.95
	1.00	c							
JICAMA (YAMBEAN)									
raw	100.00	g	38	0.7	8.8	4.00	150.0	18.00	0.09
	86.67	g	33	0.6	7.6	3.47	130.0	15.60	0.08
	0.67	c							
boiled, drained, no salt 1 svg= 3oz	100.00	g	38	0.7	8.8	4.00	135.0	16.00	0.09
	85.05	g	32	0.6	7.5	3.40	114.8	13.61	0.08
	3.00	oz							

ARUGULA	SERVING QUANTITY	SERVING UNIT	CALORIES (kCal)	PROTEIN (g)	TOTAL CARBOHYDRATES (g)	SODIUM (mg)	POTASSIUM (mg)	PHOSPHORUS (mg)	TOTAL FAT (g)
raw, leaves	100	g	25	2.6	3.7	27.00	369	52.00	0.66
	80.00	g	20	2.1	2.9	21.60	295	41.60	0.53
	4.00	c							
salad mixed	100	g	18	1.5	3.3	16.94	299	32.15	0.27
baby greens	41.25	g	7	0.6	1.4	6.99	123	13.26	0.11
Arugula,butterhead, endives, Radicchio	1.00	c							
ENDIVE OR ESCAROLE									
raw, chopped	100	g	17	1.3	3.4	22.00	314.0	28.00	0.20
	87.50	g	15	1.1	2.9	19.25	274.7	24.50	0.18
	1.75	c							
Chicory, Witlof	100	g	17	0.9	4.0	2.00	211.0	26.00	0.10
or Belgium	90.00	g	15	0.8	3.6	1.80	189.9	23.40	0.09
	1.00	c							
OKRA									
raw	100	g	33	1.9	7.5	7.00	299.0	61.00	0.19
	75.00	g	25	1.5	5.6	5.25	224.2	45.75	0.14
	0.75	c							
sliced, boiled,	100	g	22	1.9	4.5	6.00	135.0	32.00	0.21
drained, n.s.	80.00	g	18	1.5	3.6	4.80	108.0	25.60	0.17
	0.50	c							
frozen	100	g	30	1.7	6.6	3.00	211.0	42.00	0.25
	85.05	g	26	1.4	5.6	2.55	179.4	35.72	0.21
	3.00	oz							
frozen, boiled,	100	g	29	1.6	6.4	3.00	184.0	37.00	0.24
drained, no salt	92.00	g	27	1.5	5.9	2.76	169.2	34.04	0.22
sliced	0.50	c							
PUMPKIN									
fruit/meat, raw,	100	g	26	1.0	6.5	1.00	340.0	44.00	0.10
cut 1" cube	116	g	30	1.2	7.5	1.16	394.4	51.04	0.12
	1.00	c							
boiled, drained,	100	g	20	0.7	4.9	1.00	230.0	30.00	0.07
mashed, n.s.	122.5	g	25	0.9	6.0	1.23	281.7	36.75	0.09
	0.50	c							
flowers	100	g	15	0.0	3.3	5.00	173.0	49.00	0.07
	33.00	g	1	0.0	0.1	0.20	6.92	1.96	0.00
	1.00	c							
flowers, boiled,	100	g	15	1.1	3.3	6.00	106.0	34.00	0.08
drained	89.33	g	13	1.0	3.0	5.36	5.36	30.37	0.07
	0.67	c							
seeds (squash	100	g	559	30.2	10.7	7.00	809.0	1,233	49.05
kernels), dried	34.50	g	193	10.4	3.7	2.42	279.1	425.4	16.92
	0.25	c							
seeds	100	g	446	18.6	53.8	18.00	919.0	92.00	19.40
(pumkin/squash), whole,	32.00	g	143	5.9	17.2	5.76	294.0	29.44	6.21
roasted no salt added	0.50	c							

SQUASH	SERVING QUANTITY	SERVING UNIT	CALORIES (kCal)	PROTEIN (g)	TOTAL CARBOHYDRATES (g)	SODIUM (mg)	POTASSIUM (mg)	PHOSPHORUS (mg)	TOTAL FAT (g)
winter,	100.00	g	34	1.0	8.6	4.00	350.0	23.00	0.13
all varieties cubes	116.00	g	39	1.1	10.0	4.64	406.0	26.68	0.15
	1.00	c							
butternut	100.00	g	45	1.0	11.7	4.00	352.0	33.00	0.10
cubes	140.00	g	63	1.4	16.4	5.60	492.8	46.20	0.14
	1.00	c							
winter,	100.00	g	57	1.8	14.4	2.00	212.0	22.00	0.10
butternut, frozen	85.05	g	48	1.5	12.3	1.70	180.3	18.71	0.09
	3.00	oz							
summer,	100.00	g	16	1.2	3.4	2.00	262.0	38.00	0.18
all varieties sliced	84.75	g	14	1.0	2.8	1.70	222.0	32.21	0.15
	0.75	c							
KOHLRABI									
raw	100.00	g	27	1.7	6.2	20.00	350.0	46.00	0.10
	135.00	g	36	2.3	8.4	27.00	472.5	62.10	0.14
	1.00	c							
boiled,	100.00	g	29	1.8	6.7	21.00	340.0	45.00	0.11
drained, sliced	165.00	g	48	3.0	11.0	34.65	561.0	74.25	0.18
	1.00	c							
LEEKS									
raw	100.00	g	61	1.5	14.2	20.00	180.0	35.00	0.30
	89.00	g	54	1.3	12.6	17.80	160.2	31.15	0.27
	1.00	c							
boiled, drained,	100.00	g	31	0.8	7.6	10.00	87.00	17.00	0.20
chopped or diced	26.00	g	8	0.2	2.0	2.60	22.62	4.42	0.05
	0.25	c							
CASSAVA/YUCCA/MANIOC									
raw	100.00	g	160	1.4	38.1	14.00	271.0	27.00	0.28
	103.00	g	165	1.4	39.2	14.42	279.1	27.81	0.29
	0.50	c							
RADISH									
oriental (Daikon),	100.00	g	18	0.6	4.1	21.00	227.0	23.00	0.10
7" long	338.00	g	61	2.0	13.9	70.98	767.2	77.74	0.34
	1.00	pc							
oriental, boiled,	100.00	g	17	0.7	3.4	13.00	285.0	24.00	0.24
drained, no salt sliced	73.50	g	13	0.5	2.5	9.56	209.5	17.64	0.18
	0.50	c							
sprouts	100.00	g	43	3.8	3.6	6.00	86.00	113.0	2.53
	38.00	g	16	1.5	1.4	2.28	32.68	42.94	0.96
	1.00	c							

	SERVING QUANTITY	SERVING UNIT	CALORIES (kCal)	PROTEIN (g)	TOTAL CARBOHYDRATES (g)	SODIUM (mg)	POTASSIUM (mg)	PHOSPHORUS (mg)	TOTAL FAT (g)
SWISS CHARD									
raw	100.00	g	19	1.8	3.7	213.0	379.0	46.00	0.20
	36.00	g	7	0.7	1.4	76.68	136.4	16.56	0.07
	1.00	c							
boiled, drained, no salt	100.00	g	20	1.9	4.1	179.0	549.0	33.00	0.08
	175.00	g	35	3.3	7.2	313.2	960.7	57.75	0.14
	1.00	c							
SPINACH									
raw, chopped	100.00	g	23	2.9	3.6	79.00	558.0	49.00	0.39
	90.00	g	21	2.6	3.3	71.10	502.2	44.10	0.35
	3.00	c							
frozen	100.00	g	29	3.6	4.2	74.00	346.0	49.00	0.57
	78.00	g	23	2.8	3.3	57.72	269.8	38.22	0.44
	0.50	c							
chopped, boiled, drained, no salt	100.00	g	23	3.0	3.8	70.00	466.0	56.00	0.26
	90.00	g	21	2.7	3.4	63.00	419.4	50.40	0.23
	0.50	c							
mustard (Tendergreens)	100.00	g	22	2.2	3.9	21.00	449.0	28.00	0.30
	150.00	g	33	3.3	5.9	31.50	673.5	42.00	0.45
	1.00	c							
mustard, boiled, drained, no salt	100.00	g	16	1.7	2.8	14.00	285.0	18.00	0.20
	180.00	g	29	3.1	5.0	25.20	513.0	32.40	0.36
	1.00	c							
TOMATILLOS									
chopped	100.00	g	32	1.0	5.8	1.00	268.0	39.00	1.02
	132.00	g	42	1.3	7.7	1.32	353.7	51.48	1.35
	1.00	c							
TURNIPS									
raw	100.00	g	28	0.9	6.4	67.00	191.0	27.00	0.10
	130.00	g	34	1.1	7.8	81.74	233.0	32.94	0.12
	1.00	c							
frozen	100.00	g	16	1.0	2.9	25.00	137.0	20.00	0.16
	85.05	g	14	0.9	2.5	21.26	116.5	17.01	0.14
	3.00	oz							
cubed, boiled, drained, no salt	100.00	g	22	0.7	5.1	16.00	177.0	40.56	0.08
	156.00	g	34	1.1	7.9	24.96	276.1	26.00	0.12
	1.00	c							
frozen, boiled, drained, no salt	100.00	g	23	1.5	4.4	36.00	182.0	26.00	0.24
	78.00	g	18	1.2	3.4	28.08	142	20.28	0.19
	0.50	c							

TURNIP GREENS	SERVING QUANTITY	SERVING UNIT	CALORIES (kCal)	PROTEIN (g)	TOTAL CARBOHYDRATES (g)	SODIUM (mg)	POTASSIUM (mg)	PHOSPHORUS (mg)	TOTAL FAT (g)
raw, turnip greens, chopped	100.00	g	32	1.5	7.1	40.00	296.0	42.00	0.30
	82.50	g	26	1.2	5.9	33.00	244.2	34.65	0.25
	1.50	c							
frozen	100.00	g	22	2.5	3.7	12.00	184.0	27.00	0.31
	82.00	g	18	2.0	3.0	9.84	150.8	22.14	0.25
	0.50	c							
canned	100.00	g	14	1.4	2.4	277.0	141.0	21.00	0.30
	78.00	g	11	1.1	1.9	216.0	110.0	16.38	0.23
	0.33	c							
chopped, boiled, drained, no salt	100.00	g	20	1.1	4.4	29.00	203.0	29.00	0.23
	144.00	g	29	1.6	6.3	41.76	292.3	41.76	0.33
	1.00	c							
canned, with no salt	100.00	g	19	1.4	2.8	29.00	141.0	21.00	0.30
	144.00	g	27	2.0	4.1	41.76	203.0	30.24	0.43
	1.00	c							
frozen, chopped, boiled, drained, no salt added	100.00	g	29	3.4	5.0	15.00	224.0	34.00	0.42
	164.00	g	48	5.5	8.2	24.60	367.3	55.76	0.69
	1.00	c							
RUTABAGA									
raw, cubes	100.00	g	37	1.1	8.6	12.00	305.0	53.00	0.16
	93.33	g	35	1.0	8.1	11.20	284.6	49.47	0.15
	0.67	c							
boiled, drained, no salt cubed	100.00	g	30	0.9	6.8	5.00	216.0	41.00	0.18
	170.00	g	51	1.6	11.6	8.50	367.2	69.70	0.31
	1.00	c							
boiled, drained, mashed	100.00	g	30	0.9	6.8	5.00	216.0	41.00	0.18
	160.80	g	48	1.5	11.0	8.04	347.3	65.93	0.29
	0.67	c							
PARSNIPS									
raw, sliced	100.00	g	75	1.2	18.0	10.00	375.0	71.00	0.30
	88.67	g	67	1.1	16.0	8.87	332.5	62.95	0.27
	0.67	c							
boiled, drained, sliced, no salt	100.00	g	71	1.3	17.0	10.00	367.0	69.00	0.30
	78.00	g	55	1.0	13.3	7.80	286.2	53.82	0.23
	0.50	c							

WATER CHESTNUTS	SERVING QUANTITY	SERVING UNIT	CALORIES (kCal)	PROTEIN (g)	TOTAL CARBOHYDRATES (g)	SODIUM (mg)	POTASSIUM (mg)	PHOSPHORUS (mg)	TOTAL FAT (g)
fresh, raw, Chinese (Matai) slices	100.00	g	97	1.4	23.9	14.00	584.0	63.00	0.10
	62.00	g	60	0.9	14.8	8.68	362.0	39.06	0.06
	0.50	c							
canned with liquid Chinese (Matai)	100.00	g	50	0.9	12.3	8.00	118.0	19.00	0.06
	70.00	g	35	0.6	8.6	5.60	82.60	13.30	0.04
	0.50	c							
WATERCRESS									
raw, chopped	100.00	g	11	2.3	1.3	41.00	330.0	60.00	0.10
	34.00	g	4	0.8	0.4	13.94	112.2	20.40	0.03
	1.00	c							
YAM									
raw, in cubes	100.00	g	118	1.5	28.0	9.00	816.0	55.00	0.17
	112.50	g	133	1.7	31.4	10.13	918.0	61.88	0.19
	0.75	c							
baked or broiled, drained, no salt cubed	100.00	g	116	1.5	27.5	8.00	670.0	49.00	0.14
	68.00	g	79	1.0	18.7	5.44	455.6	33.32	0.10
	0.50	c							
Hawaiian Mountain, raw cubed	100.00	g	67	1.3	16.3	13.00	418.0	34.00	0.10
	68.00	g	46	0.9	11.1	8.84	284.2	23.12	0.07
	0.50	c							
Hawaiian Mountain, steamed cubed	100.00	g	82	1.7	20.0	12.00	495.0	40.00	0.08
	145.00	g	119	2.5	29.0	17.40	717.7	58.00	0.12
	1.00	c							
MIXED VEGETABLES									
frozen	100.00	g	72	3.3	13.5	47.00	212.0	59.00	0.52
	72.00	g	52	2.4	9.7	33.84	152.6	42.48	0.37
	0.50	c							
frozen, boiled, drained, no salt added	100.00	g	65	2.9	13.1	35.00	169.0	51.00	0.15
	91.00	g	59	2.6	11.9	31.85	153.8	46.41	0.14
	0.50	c							
canned, drained	100.00	g	49	2.6	9.3	214.0	291.0	42.00	0.25
	163.00	g	80	4.2	15.1	348.8	474.3	68.46	0.41
	1.00	c							
BRUSSEL SPROUTS									
raw	100.00	g	43	33.4	9.0	25.00	389.0	69.00	0.30
	88.00	g	38	3.0	7.9	22.00	342.0	60.70	0.26
	1.00	c							

KALE	SERVING QUANTITY	SERVING UNIT	CALORIES (kCal)	PROTEIN (g)	TOTAL CARBOHYDRATES (g)	SODIUM (mg)	POTASSIUM (mg)	PHOSPHORUS (mg)	TOTAL FAT (g)
raw, chopped	100.00	g	35	2.9	4.4	53.00	348.0	55.00	1.49
	83.75	g	29	2.5	3.7	44.39	291.4	46.06	1.25
	1.25	c							
chopped, boiled,	100.00	g	36	2.9	5.3	16.00	144.0	42.00	1.21
drained, no salt	65.00	g	23	1.9	3.5	10.40	93.60	27.30	0.79
	0.50	c							
scotch, raw,	100.00	g	42	2.8	8.3	70.00	450.0	62.00	0.60
chopped	83.75	g	35	2.4	7.0	58.63	376.8	51.93	0.50
	1.25	c							
scotch, boiled,	100.00	g	28	1.9	5.6	45.00	274.0	38.00	0.41
drained, chopped no salt	86.67	g	24	1.7	4.9	39.00	237.4	32.93	0.36
	0.67	c							
frozen, raw	100.00	g	28	2.7	4.9	15.00	333.0	29.00	0.46
1 pack=10 oz/ 284g	85.05	g	24	2.3	4.2	12.76	283.2	24.66	0.39
	3.00	oz							
frozen, chopped,	100.00	g	36	2.9	5.3	16.00	144.0	42.00	1.21
boiled, drained, no salt	65.00	g	23	1.9	3.5	10.40	93.60	27.30	0.79
	0.50	c							
MUSTARD GREENS									
raw, chopped	100.00	g	27	2.9	4.7	20.00	384.0	58.00	0.42
	84.00	g	23	2.4	3.9	16.80	322.5	48.72	0.35
	1.50	c							
boiled, drained,	100.00	g	26	2.6	4.5	9.00	162.0	42.00	0.47
chopped, no salt	70.00	g	18	1.8	3.2	6.30	113.4	29.40	0.33
	0.50	c							
frozen	100.00	g	20	2.5	3.4	29.00	170.0	30.00	0.27
1 pack=10oz/284g	73.00	g	15	1.8	2.5	21.17	124.1	21.90	0.20
	0.50	c							
frozen, boiled,	100.00	g	19	2.3	3.1	25.00	139.0	24.00	0.25
drained, no salt 1 pack = 10oz/ 212g	75.00	g	14	1.7	2.3	18.75	104.2	18.00	0.19
	0.50	c							

B. Vegetable Proteins

Hey there!

Do you need to print out this Food List?

You can download a printable version of this chart by scanning the QR code below or copying the link on your computer browser.

https://go.renaltracker.com/printfoodlist

BEANS

BEANS	SERVING QUANTITY	SERVING UNIT	CALORIES (kCal)	PROTEIN (g)	TOTAL CARBOHYDRATES (g)	SODIUM (mg)	POTASSIUM (mg)	PHOSPHORUS (mg)	TOTAL FAT (g)
Lentils/Pinto/	100.00	g	131	8.6	23.9	1.67	398.9	165.7	0.49
Navy	92.00	g	121	8.0	22.0	1.54	367.0	152.5	0.45
	0.50	c							
Lima	100.00	g	113	6.8	20.2	8.00	467.0	136.0	0.86
	78.00	g	88	5.3	15.7	6.24	364.2	106.0	0.67
	0.50	c							
Broad or Fava	100.00	g	72	5.6	11.7	50.00	250.0	95.00	0.60
	81.75	g	59	4.6	9.6	40.88	204.3	77.60	0.49
	0.75	c							
Black beans,	100.00	g	132	8.9	23.7	1.00	355.0	140.0	0.54
boiled	86.00	g	114	7.6	20.4	0.86	305.3	120.4	0.46
	0.50	c							
Mungo,	100.00	g	105	7.5	18.3	7.00	231.0	156.0	0.55
boiled	90.00	g	95	6.8	16.5	6.30	207.9	140.4	0.50
	0.50	c							
sprouts, Mung	100.00	g	30	3.0	5.9	6.00	149.0	54.00	0.18
	78.00	g	23	2.4	4.6	4.68	116.2	42.12	0.14
	0.75	c							
Kidney, boiled	100.00	g	127	8.7	22.8	1.00	405.0	138.0	0.50
	88.50	g	112	7.7	20.2	0.89	358.4	122.1	0.44
	0.50	c							
Navy, boiled	100.00	g	140	8.2	26.1	0.00	389.0	144.0	0.62
	91.00	g	127	7.5	23.7	0.00	354.0	131.0	0.56
	0.50	c							
Lupin, boiled	100.00	g	119	15	9.9	4.00	245.0	128.0	2.92
	83.00	g	99	12	8.2	3.32	203.3	106.2	2.42
	0.50	c							
Pinto, frozen	100.00	g	170	9.8	32.5	92.00	755.9	117.0	0.50
	94.49	g	161	9.3	31.0	86.93	714.3	110.5	0.47
	3.33	Oz							
Pinto, boiled	100.00	g	143	9.0	26.2	1.00	436.0	147.0	0.65
	85.50	g	122	7.7	22.4	0.86	372.8	125.7	0.56
	0.50	c							
White	100.00	g	139	9.7	25.1	6.00	561.0	113.0	0.35
(Cannellini), boiled no salt	89.50	g	124	8.7	22.5	5.37	502.1	101.1	0.31
	0.50	c							

BEANS

BEANS	Serving Quantity	Serving Unit	Calories (kCal)	Protein (g)	Total Carbohydrates (g)	Sodium (mg)	Potassium (mg)	Phosphorus (mg)	Total Fat (g)
White, small, boiled, no salt	100.00	g	142	9.0	25.8	2.00	463.0	169.0	0.64
	89.50	g	127	8.0	23.1	1.79	414.4	151.2	0.57
	0.50	c							
sprouts, Kidney	100.00	g	29	4.2	4.1	6.00	187.0	37.00	0.50
	92.00	g	27	3.9	3.8	5.52	172.0	34.04	0.46
	0.50	c							
Sprouts, Navy	100.00	g	67	6.2	13.1	13.00	307.0	100.0	0.70
	78.00	g	52	4.8	10.2	10.14	239.4	78.00	0.55
	0.75	c							
sprouts, Pinto	100.00	g	62	5.3	11.6	153.0	307.0	94.00	0.90
	85.05	g	53	4.5	9.9	130.1	262.1	79.95	0.77
	3.00	oz							
French, boiled	100.00	g	129	7.1	24.0	6.00	370.0	102.0	0.76
	88.50	g	114	6.2	21.3	5.31	327.4	90.27	0.67
	0.50	c							
baked, prepared	100.00	g	155	5.5	21.6	422.0	358.0	109.0	5.15
	126.50	g	196	7.0	27.4	533.8	452.8	138.0	6.51
	0.50	c							
Refried, canned	100.00	g	90	5.0	13.6	370.0	319.0	92.00	2.01
	119.00	g	107	5.9	16.1	440.3	379.6	109.4	2.39
	0.50	c							

CHICKPEAS

CHICKPEAS	Serving Quantity	Serving Unit	Calories (kCal)	Protein (g)	Total Carbohydrates (g)	Sodium (mg)	Potassium (mg)	Phosphorus (mg)	Total Fat (g)
garbanzos/ Bengal gram, canned	100.00	g	88	4.9	13.5	278.0	144.0	80.00	1.95
	120.00	g	106	5.9	16.2	333.6	172.8	96.00	2.34
	0.50	c							
garbanzos/ Bengal gram, boiled	100.00	g	164	8.9	27.4	7.00	291.0	168.0	2.59
	82.00	g	134	7.3	22.5	5.74	238.6	137.7	2.12
	0.50	c							
garbanzos/ Bengal gram, canned drained, rinsed in tap water	100.00	g	138	7.0	22.9	212.0	109.0	80.00	2.47
	152.00	g	210	10.7	34.8	322.3	165.6	121.6	3.75
	1.00	c							
garbanzos/ Bengal gram, canned low sodium	100	g	88	4.9	13.5	132.0	144.0	80.00	1.95
	240	g	211	11.8	32.4	316.8	345.6	192.0	4.68
	1	c							
flour	100.00	g	387	22.4	57.8	64.00	846.0	318.0	6.69
	92.00	g	110	6.4	16.4	18.14	239.8	90.15	1.90
	1.00	c							

	SERVING QUANTITY	SERVING UNIT	CALORIES (kCal)	PROTEIN (g)	TOTAL CARBOHYDRATES (g)	SODIUM (mg)	POTASSIUM (mg)	PHOSPHORUS (mg)	TOTAL FAT (g)
TOFU									
soft with calcium sulfate and magnesium chloride (Nigari)	100.00	g	61	7.2	1.2	8.00	120.0	92.00	3.69
	85.05	g	52	6.1	1.0	6.80	102.0	78.25	3.14
	3.00	oz							
firm with calcium sulfate and magnesium chloride (Nigari)	100.00	g	78	9.0	2.9	12.00	148.0	121.0	4.17
	85.05	g	66	7.7	2.4	10.21	125.8	102.9	3.55
	3.00	oz							
silken tofu (Vitasoy USA)	100.00	g	43	4.8	0.6	2.00	Na	na	2.40
	91.00	g	39	4.4	0.5	1.82	Na	na	2.18
	0.20	Package							
TEMPEH									
raw	100.00	g	192	20.3	7.6	9.00	412.0	266.0	10.80
	83.00	g	159	16.8	6.3	7.47	341.9	220.8	8.96
	0.50	c							
cooked	100.00	g	185	19.8	7.6	14.00	401.0	253.0	11.38
EDAMAME									
frozen, unprepared	100.00	g	109	11.2	7.6	6.00	482.0	161.0	4.73
	118.00	g	129	13.2	9.0	7.08	568.7	189.9	5.58
	1.00	c							
frozen, prepared	100.00	g	121	11.9	8.9	6.00	436.0	261.9	5.20
	155.00	g	188	18.5	13.8	9.30	676	169	8.06
	1.00	c							
SPIRULINA									
seaweed, fresh/ raw	100.00	g	26	5.9	2.4	98.00	127	11.00	0.39
	28.35	g	7	1.7	0.7	27.78	36.00	3.12	0.11
	1.00	Oz							
seaweed, dried	100.00	g	290	57.5	23.9	1,048	1363	118	7.72
	112.00	g	325	64.4	26.8	1,174	1527	133	8.65
	1.00	c							

C. Fruits

Hey there!

Do you need to print out this Food List?

You can download a printable version of this chart by scanning the QR code below or copying the link on your computer browser.

https://go.renaltracker.com/printfoodlist

APPLE

	SERVING QUANTITY	SERVING UNIT	CALORIES (KCal)	PROTEIN (g)	TOTAL CARBOHYDRATES (g)	SODIUM (mg)	POTASSIUM (mg)	PHOSPHORUS (mg)	TOTAL FAT (g)
Gala, raw, with skin	100.0	g	57	0.3	13.7	1.00	108.0	11.00	0.12
	172.0	g	98	0.4	23.5	1.72	185.7	18.92	0.21
	1.00	pc, med							
fuji, raw, with skin	100.0	g	63	0.2	15.2	1.00	109.0	13.00	0.18
	192.0	g	121	0.4	29.2	1.92	209.2	24.96	0.35
	1.00	pc, med							
golden delicious, with skin	100.0	g	57	0.3	13.6	2.00	100.0	10.00	0.15
	169.0	g	96	0.5	23.0	3.38	169.0	16.90	0.25
	1.00	pc, med							
granny smith, w/ skin, raw	100.0	g	58	0.4	13.6	1.00	120.0	12.00	0.19
	167.0	g	97	0.7	22.7	1.67	200.4	20.04	0.32
	1.00	pc, med							
juice, frozen concentrate	100.0	g	47	0.1	11.5	7.00	126.0	7.00	0.10
	239.0	g	112	0.3	27.6	16.73	301.1	16.73	0.24
	8.00	fl oz							
applesauce, sweetened, canned	100.0	g	68	0.2	17.5	2.00	75.00	6.00	0.17
	123.0	g	84	0.2	21.5	2.46	92.25	7.38	0.21
	0.50	c							
applesauce, unsweetened, canned	100.0	g	42	0.2	11.3	2.00	74.00	5.00	0.10
	122.0	g	51	0.2	13.8	2.44	90.28	6.10	0.12
	0.50	c							

BLACK BERRIES

	SERVING QUANTITY	SERVING UNIT	CALORIES (KCal)	PROTEIN (g)	TOTAL CARBOHYDRATES (g)	SODIUM (mg)	POTASSIUM (mg)	PHOSPHORUS (mg)	TOTAL FAT (g)
raw	100.0	g	43	1.4	9.6	1.00	162.0	22.00	0.49
	144.0	g	62	2.0	13.8	1.44	233.2	31.68	0.71
	1.00	c							
frozen, unsweetened	100.0	g	64	1.2	15.7	1.00	140.0	30.00	0.43
	151.0	g	97	1.8	23.7	1.51	211.4	45.30	0.65
	1.00	c							
canned, heavy syrup	100.0	g	92	1.3	23.1	3.00	99.00	14.00	0.14
	256.0	g	236	3.4	59.1	7.68	253.4	35.84	0.36
	1.00	c							

RASP BERRIES	SERVING QUANTITY	SERVING UNIT	CALORIES (kCal)	PROTEIN (g)	TOTAL CARBOHYDRATES (g)	SODIUM (mg)	POTASSIUM (mg)	PHOSPHORUS (mg)	TOTAL FAT (g)
raw	100.0	g	52	1.2	11.9	1.00	151.0	29.00	0.69
	123.0	g	64	1.5	14.7	1.23	185.7	35.67	0.80
	1.00	c							
frozen, unsweetened	100.0	g	56	1.2	12.6	4.00	184.0	30.00	0.81
	140.0	g	78	1.6	17.6	5.60	257.6	42.00	1.13
	1.00	c							
red, frozen, sweetened, unthawed	100.0	g	103	0.7	26.2	1.00	114.0	17.00	0.16
	125.0	g	129	0.9	32.7	1.25	142.5	21.25	0.20
	0.50	c							
puree, with seeds	100.0	g	55	na	11.5	4.00	195.0	30.00	0.97
juice concentrate	100.0	g	221	3.0	53.2	10.0	1,178	100.0	1.34
PEARS									
whole, medium (2.5/lb)	100.0	g	57	0.4	15.2	1.00	116.0	16.00	0.14
	166.0	g	95	0.6	25.3	1.66	192.5	19.92	0.23
	1.00	pc							
halves, canned in water	100.0	g	29	0.2	7.8	2.00	53.00	7.00	0.03
	244.0	g	71	0.5	19.1	4.88	129.3	17.08	0.07
	1.00	c							
Asian	100.0	g	42	0.5	10.7	0.00	121.0	11.00	0.23
	122.0	g	51	0.6	13.0	0.00	147.6	13.42	0.28
	1.00	pc							
CRANBERRY									
fresh, chopped	100.0	g	46	0.5	12.0	2.00	80.00	11.00	0.13
	55.00	g	25	0.3	6.6	1.10	44.00	6.05	0.07
	0.50	c							
dried, sweetened	100.0	g	308	0.2	82.8	5.00	49.00	8.00	1.09
	40.00	g	123	0.1	33.1	2.00	19.60	3.20	0.44
	0.33	c							
juice, unsweetened	100.0	g	46	0.4	12.2	2.00	77.00	13.00	0.13
	253.0	g	116	1.0	30.9	5.06	194.8	32.89	0.33
	1.00	c							
juice, cran cocktail	100.0	g	54	0.0	13.5	2.00	14.00	1.00	0.10
	253.0	g	137	0.0	34.2	5.06	35.42	2.53	0.25
	8.00	fl oz							
sauce, canned, sweetened	100.0	g	159	0.9	40.4	5.00	28.00	4.00	0.15
	69.25	g	110	0.6	28.0	3.46	19.39	2.77	0.10
	0.25	c							

GRAPE

GRAPE	SERVING QUANTITY	SERVING UNIT	CALORIES (kCal)	PROTEIN (g)	TOTAL CARBOHYDRATES (g)	SODIUM (mg)	POTASSIUM (mg)	PHOSPHORUS (mg)	TOTAL FAT (g)
red or green, seedless	100.0	g	69	0.7	18.1	2.00	191.0	20.00	0.16
	151.0	g	104	1.1	27.3	3.02	288.4	30.20	0.24
	1.00	c							
juice, unsweetened, plus Vit.C	100.0	g	60	0.4	14.8	5.00	104.0	14.00	0.13
	252.8	g	152	0.9	37.3	12.64	262.9	35.39	0.33
	8.00	fl oz							
fruit mixed/ fruit cocktail, light, drained	100.0	g	55	0.4	14.3	6.00	85.00	13.00	0.08
juice, sweetened, frozen concentrate 6 fl oz can	100.0	g	179	0.7	44.4	7.00	74.00	15.00	0.31
	216.0	g	387	1.4	95.8	15.12	159.8	32.40	0.67
	1.00	can/ item							
seedless, Thompson, canned in water	100.0	g	40	0.5	10.3	6.00	107.0	18.00	0.11
	245.0	g	98	1.2	25.2	14.70	262.1	44.10	0.27
	1.00	c							
jelly 1 packet= 14g (0.5oz)	100.0	g	266	0.2	70.0	30.00	54.00	6.00	0.02
	21.00	g	56	0.0	14.7	6.30	11.34	1.26	0.00
	1	tbsp							

PINE APPLE

	SERVING QUANTITY	SERVING UNIT	CALORIES (kCal)	PROTEIN (g)	TOTAL CARBOHYDRATES (g)	SODIUM (mg)	POTASSIUM (mg)	PHOSPHORUS (mg)	TOTAL FAT (g)
traditional varieties, diced	100.0	g	45	0.6	18.3	1.00	125.0	9.00	0.13
	155.0	g	70	0.9	11.8	1.55	193.7	13.95	0.20
	1.00	c							
sweetened, frozen, chunks	100.0	g	86	0.4	22.2	2.00	100.0	4.00	0.10
	245.0	g	211	1.0	54.4	4.90	245.0	9.80	0.25
	1.00	c							
canned in water crushed, sliced, or chunks	100.0	g	32	0.4	8.3	1.00	127.0	4.00	0.09
	246.0	g	79	1.1	20.4	2.46	312.4	9.84	0.22
	1.00	c							
canned in juice crushed, sliced, or chunks	100.0	g	60	0.4	15.7	1.00	122.0	6.00	0.08
	249.0	g	149	1.1	39.1	2.49	303.8	14.94	0.20
	1.00	c							
extra sweet variety, diced	100.0	g	51	0.5	13.5	1.00	108.0	8.00	0.11
	155.0	g	79	0.8	20.9	1.55	167.4	12.40	0.17
	1.00	c							
juice, unsweetened, canned	100.0	g	53	0.4	12.9	2.00	130.0	8.00	0.12
	250.0	g	133	0.9	32.2	5.00	325.0	20.00	0.30
	8.00	fl oz							
canned in light syrup crushed, sliced, or chunks	100.0	g	52	0.4	13.5	1.00	105.0	7.00	0.12
	126.0	g	66	0.5	17.0	1.26	132.3	8.82	0.15
	0.50	c							
juice, unsweetened, frozen concentrate	100.0	g	179	1.3	44.3	3.00	472.0	28.00	0.10
	288.0	g	387	2.8	95.7	6.48	1,019	60.48	0.22
	1.00	c							
juice, 55pprox.55ned with Vit A, C & E	100.0	g	50	0.4	12.2	3.00	132.0	9.00	0.14
	250.0	g	125	0.9	30.5	7.50	330.0	22.50	0.35
	1.00	c							

BLUE BERRIES	SERVING QUANTITY	SERVING UNIT	CALORIES (kCal)	PROTEIN (g)	TOTAL CARBOHYDRATES (g)	SODIUM (mg)	POTASSIUM (mg)	PHOSPHORUS (mg)	TOTAL FAT (g)
fresh	100.0	g	57	0.7	14.5	1.00	77.00	12.00	0.33
	145.0	g	83	1.1	21.0	1.45	111.6	17.40	0.48
	1.00	c							
sweetened,	100.0	g	317	2.5	80.0	3.00	214.0	36.00	2.50
dried	40.00	g	127	1.0	32.0	1.20	85.60	14.40	1.00
	0.25	c							
wild, frozen	100.0	g	57	0.0	13.9	3.00	68.00	13.00	0.16
	140.0	g	80	0.0	19.4	4.20	95.20	18.20	0.22
	1.00	c							
unsweetened,	100.0	g	51	0.4	12.2	1.00	54.00	11.00	0.64
frozen	155.0	g	79	0.7	18.9	1.55	83.70	17.05	0.99
	1.00	c							
canned, light	100.0	g	88	1.0	22.7	3.00	54.00	12.00	0.40
syrup , drained	244.0	g	215	2.5	55.3	7.32	131.7	29.28	0.98
	1.00	c							
STRAWBERRIES									
fresh, whole	100.0	g	32	0.7	7.7	1.00	153.0	24.00	0.30
	144.0	g	46	1.0	11.1	1.44	220.3	34.56	0.43
	1.00	c							
unsweetened,	100.0	g	35	0.4	9.1	2.00	148.0	13.00	0.11
frozen	149.0	g	52	0.6	13.6	2.98	220.5	19.37	
(unthawed)									0.16
	1.00	c							
sweetened,	100.0	g	78	0.5	21.0	1.00	98.00	12.00	0.14
frozen, thawed	127.5	g	99	0.7	26.8	1.28	124.9	15.30	0.18
	0.50	c							
fruit topping	100.0	g	254	0.2	66.3	21.00	51.00	5.00	0.10
	42.00	g	107	0.1	27.9	8.82	21.42	2.10	0.04
	2.00	tbsp							
pastry,	100.0	g	371	5.4	47.8	445.0	83.00	89.00	18.50
56pprox,	71.00	g	263	3.8	33.9	315.9	58.93	63.19	13.14
enriched									
	1.00	pc							
Milkshake	100.0	g	113	3.4	18.9	83.00	182.0	100.0	2.80
(fastfood)	226.4	g	256	7.7	42.8	187.9	412.1	226.4	6.34
	8.00	fl oz							
yogurt 56ppro,	100.0	g	105	8.2	12.3	33.00	129.0	109.0	2.57
low fat									
1 item = 1	150.0	g	158	12.3	18.4	49.50	193.5	163.5	3.86
container									
	1.00	item							

GRAPEFRUIT	SERVING QUANTITY	SERVING UNIT	CALORIES (kCal)	PROTEIN (g)	TOTAL CARBOHYDRATES (g)	SODIUM (mg)	POTASSIUM (mg)	PHOSPHORUS (mg)	TOTAL FAT (g)
fresh	100.0	g	32	0.6	8.1	0.00	139.0	8.00	0.10
	153.3	g	49	1.0	12.4	0.00	213.1	12.27	0.15
	0.67	c							
white, fresh,	100.0	g	33	0.7	8.4	0.00	148.0	8.00	0.10
small (3.5 diameter)	118.0	g	39	0.8	9.9	0.00	174.6	9.44	0.12
	0.50	Pc							
pink or red	100.0	g	42	0.8	10.7	0.00	135.0	18.00	0.14
	153.3	g	64	1.2	16.4	0.00	207.0	27.60	0.21
	0.67	c							
juice, white	100.0	g	39	0.5	9.2	1.00	162.0	15.00	0.10
	247.0	g	96	1.2	22.7	2.47	400.2	37.05	0.25
	8.00	fl oz							
juice, pink	100.0	g	39	0.5	9.2	1.00	162.0	15.00	0.10
	247.0	g	96	1.2	22.7	2.47	400.2	37.05	0.25
	1.00	c							
juice,	100.0	g	37	0.6	7.5	2.00	141.0	17.00	0.66
unsweetened, pink, canned	247.2	g	91	1.4	18.6	4.94	348.6	42.02	1.63
	8.00	fl oz							
ELDERBERRIES									
	100.0	g	73	7.0	18.4	6.00	280.0	39.00	0.50
fresh	145.0	g	106	1.0	26.7	8.70	406.0	56.55	0.73
	1.00	c							
GOOSEBERRIES									
	100.0	g	44	0.9	10.2	1.00	198.0	27.00	0.58
fresh	150.0	g	66	1.3	15.3	1.50	297.0	40.50	0.87
	1.00	c							
	100.0	g	73	0.7	18.8	2.00	77.00	7.00	0.20
canned in light syrup	252.0	g	184	1.6	47.3	5.04	194.1	17.64	0.50
	1.00	c							
KIWI *(Chinese gooseberries)*									
fresh, medium,	100.0	g	61	1.1	14.7	3.00	312.0	34.00	0.52
without skin	76.00	g	46	0.9	11.1	2.28	237.1	25.84	0.40
	1.00	pc							
LOGAN BERRIES									
frozen	100.0	g	55	1.5	13.0	1.00	145.0	26.00	0.31
	147.0	g	81	2.2	19.1	1.47	213.2	38.22	0.46
	1.00	c							

CHERRIES	SERVING QUANTITY	SERVING UNIT	CALORIES (kCal)	PROTEIN (g)	TOTAL CARBOHYDRATES (g)	SODIUM (mg)	POTASSIUM (mg)	PHOSPHORUS (mg)	TOTAL FAT (g)
sweet, without pits	100.0	g	63	1.1	16.0	0.00	222.0	21.00	0.20
	154.0	g	97	1.6	24.7	0.00	341.9	32.34	0.31
	1.00	c							
sour red, without pits	100.0	g	50	1.0	12.2	3.00	173.0	15.00	0.30
	155.0	g	78	1.6	18.9	4.65	268.2	23.25	0.47
	1.00	c							
juice, tart	100.0	g	59	0.3	13.7	4.00	161.0	17.00	0.54
	269.0	g	159	0.8	36.9	10.76	433.1	45.73	1.45
	1.00	c							
Pitanga or Surinam	100.0	g	33	0.8	7.5	3.00	103.0	11.00	0.40
	173.0	g	57	1.4	13.0	5.19	178.2	19.03	0.69
	1.00	c							
tart, dried, sweetened	100.0	g	333	1.3	80.5	13.00	376.0	36.00	0.73
	40.00	g	133	0.5	32.2	5.20	150.4	14.40	0.29
	0.25	c							
maraschino, canned, drained	100.0	g	165	0.2	42.0	4.00	21.0	3.00	0.21
	5.00	g	8	0.0	2.1	0.20	1.05	0.15	0.01
	1.00	pc/ item							
sweet, canned in juice, pitted	100.0	g	54	0.9	13.8	3.00	131.0	22.00	0.02
	250.0	g	135	2.3	34.5	7.50	327.5	55.00	0.05
	1.00	c							
sweet, canned in water	100.0	g	46	0.8	11.8	1.00	131.0	15.00	0.13
	248.0	g	114	1.9	29.2	2.48	324.9	37.20	0.32
	1.00	c							
sweet, frozen, sweetened thawed	100.0	g	89	1.2	22.4	1.00	199.0	16.00	0.13
	259.0	g	231	3.0	57.9	2.59	515.4	41.44	0.34
	1.00	c							
pie filling, canned	100.0	g	115	0.4	28.0	18.00	105.0	15.00	0.07
1/8 of 21 oz can	74.00	g	85	0.3	20.7	13.32	77.70	11.10	0.05
	1.00	svg							
pie fillings, low calorie	100.0	g	53	0.8	12.0	12.00	118.0	15.00	0.16
	264.0	g	140	2.2	31.6	31.68	311.5	39.60	0.42
	1.00	c							
sour red, canned in water, drained	100.0	g	42	0.7	10.5	4.00	115.0	16.00	0.21
	168.0	g	71	1.2	17.6	6.72	193.2	26.88	0.35
	1.00	c							
sour red, 58pprox.58ned,	100.0	g	46	0.9	11.0	1.00	124.0	16.00	0.44
frozen unthawed	155.0	g	71	1.4	17.1	1.55	192.2	24.80	0.68
	1.00	c							
sour red, canned in light syrup	100.0	g	75	0.7	19.3	7.00	95.00	10.00	0.10
	126.0	g	95	0.9	24.3	8.82	119.7	12.60	0.13
	0.50	c							

PEACHES	SERVING QUANTITY	SERVING UNIT	CALORIES (kCal)	PROTEIN (g)	TOTAL CARBOHYDRATES (g)	SODIUM (mg)	POTASSIUM (mg)	PHOSPHORUS (mg)	TOTAL FAT (g)
raw, medium (59pprox. 4/lb)	100.0	g	39	0.9	9.5	0.00	190.0	20.00	0.25
	150.0	g	59	1.4	14.3	0.00	285.0	30.00	0.38
	1.00	pc/ item							
dried	100.0	g	325	4.9	83.2	10.00	1,351	162.0	1.03
	38.67	g	126	1.9	32.2	3.87	522.4	62.64	0.40
	0.33	c							
slices	100.0	g	39	0.9	9.5	0.00	190.0	20.00	0.25
	154.0	g	60	1.4	14.7	0.00	292.6	30.80	0.39
	1.00	c							
nectar, canned	100.0	g	49	0.1	11.6	11.00	30.00	3.00	0.57
	249.0	g	122	0.3	28.9	27.39	74.70	7.47	1.42
	8.00	fl oz							
pie, prepared 1/6 of 8-in. pie	100.0	g	224	1.9	33.0	217.00	125.0	22.00	10.00
	117.0	g	262	2.2	38.5	253.89	146.3	25.74	11.70
	1.00	slice							
slices, sweetened, frozen	100.0	g	94	0.6	24.0	6.00	130.0	11.00	0.13
	125.0	g	118	0.8	30.0	7.50	162.5	13.75	0.16
	0.50	c							
halves/ slices, canned in water	100.0	g	24	0.4	6.1	3.00	99.00	10.00	0.06
	122.0	g	29	0.5	7.5	3.66	120.8	12.20	0.07
	0.50	c							
halves/ slices, canned in juice	100.0	g	44	0.6	11.6	4.00	128.0	17.00	0.03
	124.0	g	55	0.8	14.4	4.96	158.7	21.08	0.04
	0.50	c							
canned in extra light syrup	100.0	g	42	0.4	11.1	5.00	74.00	11.00	0.10
	123.5	g	52	0.5	13.7	6.18	91.39	13.59	0.12
	0.50	c							
canned in heavy syrup	100.0	g	75	0.4	20.1	4.00	85.00	9.00	0.10
	242.0	g	182	1.0	48.6	9.68	205.7	21.78	0.24
	1.00	c							
canned in light syrup, drained	100.0	g	61	0.6	15.7	7.00	87.00	10.00	0.15
fruit cocktail, canned light syrup with solids and liquid	100.0	g	55	0.4	14.3	6.00	85.00	13.00	0.08

CANTALOUPE **MELON**	SERVING QUANTITY	SERVING UNIT	CALORIES (kCal)	PROTEIN (g)	TOTAL CARBOHYDRATES (g)	SODIUM (mg)	POTASSIUM (mg)	PHOSPHORUS (mg)	TOTAL FAT (g)
composite,	100.0	g	31	0.7	7.5	8.22	202.4	8.67	0.20
raw	165.5	g	51	1.1	12.5	13.60	334.9	14.34	0.33
	1.00	c							
honeydew,	100.0	g	36	0.5	9.1	18.00	228.0	11.00	0.14
balls	132.7	g	48	0.7	12.1	23.90	302.7	14.60	0.19
1 slice = 125g									
	0.75	c							
Navajo	100.0	g	21	0.8	4.1	11.00	140.0	9.00	0.20
	85.05	g	18	0.7	3.5	9.36	119.1	7.65	0.17
	3.00	oz							
melon balls,	100.0	g	33	0.8	7.9	31.00	280.0	12.00	0.25
frozen,	173.0	g	57	1.5	13.7	53.63	484.4	20.76	0.43
unthawed									
	1.00	c							

BANANA

medium, 77.8	100.0	g	89	1.1	22.8	1.00	358.0	22.00	0.33
in long	118.0	g	105	1.3	27.0	1.18	422.5	25.96	0.39
	1.00	pc/ item							
dehydrated,	100.0	g	346	3.9	88.3	3.00	1,491	74.00	1.81
powder	6.20	g	21	0.2	5.5	0.19	92.44	4.59	0.11
	1.00	tbsp							
chips, dried	100.0	g	519	2.3	58.4	6.00	536.0	56.00	14.29
	42.53	g	221	1.0	24.8	2.55	227.9	23.81	33.60
	1.50	oz							
pudding, mix	100.0	g	366	0.0	93.0	788.0	17.00	5.00	0.40
mix to make ½ c	22.00	g	81	0.0	20.5	172.3	3.74	1.10	0.09
1 package= 88g = 3 ½ oz	1.00	svg							
pudding, ready to eat	100.0	g	127	2.4	21.2	196.0	110	69.00	3.60
1 can = 5 oz	142.0	g	180	3.4	30.1	278.3	156.2	97.98	5.11
	5.00	oz							

ORANGE

ORANGE	SERVING QUANTITY	SERVING UNIT	CALORIES (KCal)	PROTEIN (g)	TOTAL CARBOHYDRATES (g)	SODIUM (mg)	POTASSIUM (mg)	PHOSPHORUS (mg)	TOTAL FAT (g)
whole, 2-5/8" diameter	100.0	g	47	0.9	11.8	0.00	181.0	14.00	0.12
	131.0	g	62	1.2	15.4	0.00	237.1	18.34	0.16
	1.00	pc/ item							
Valencia (California)	100.0	g	49	1.0	11.9	0.00	179.0	17.00	0.30
	135.0	g	66	1.4	16.1	0.00	241.7	22.95	0.41
	0.75	c							
Navel (California)	100.0	g	49	0.9	12.5	1.00	166.0	28.46	0.15
	123.7	g	61	1.1	15.5	1.24	205.4	23.00	0.19
	0.75	c							
Clementines	100.0	g	47	0.9	12.0	1.00	177.0	21.00	0.15
	74.00	g	35	0.6	8.9	0.74	130.9	15.54	0.11
	1.00	pc/ item							
orange sections	100.0	g	47	0.9	11.8	0.00	181.0	14.00	0.12
	135.0	g	63	1.3	15.9	0.00	244.4	18.90	0.16
	0.75	c							
juice	100.0	g	45	0.7	10.4	1.00	200.0	17.00	0.20
	248.0	g	112	1.7	25.8	2.48	496.0	42.16	0.50
	8.00	fl oz							
Florida, sections 1 fruit = 141g	100.0	g	46	0.7	11.5	0.00	169.0	12.00	0.21
	138.7	g	64	1.0	16.0	0.00	234.5	16.65	0.29
	0.75	c							
soda	100.0	g	48	0.0	12.3	12.00	2.00	1.00	0.00
	248.0	g	119	0.0	30.5	29.76	4.96	2.48	0.00
	8.00	fl oz							
marmalade	100.0	g	246	0.3	66.3	56.00	37.00	4.00	0.00
	20.00	g	49	0.1	13.3	11.20	7.40	0.80	0.00
	1.00	tbsp							
juice, frozen	100.0	g	95	0.5	23.2	8.00	100.0	13.00	0.00
	238.4	g	70	0.4	17.2	5.92	74.00	9.62	0.00
	1.00	c							
orange peel zest	100.0	g	97	1.5	25.0	3.00	212.0	21.00	0.20
	2.00	g	2	0.0	0.5	0.06	4.24	0.42	0.00
	1.00	tsp							
juice, unsweetened, canned	100.0	g	47	0.7	11.0	4.00	184.0	17.00	0.15
	249.0	g	117	1.7	27.4	9.96	458.2	42.33	0.37
	8.00	fl oz							
Mandarin, canned in juice	100.0	g		37	0.6	9.6	5.00	133.0	10.00
	249.0	g		92	1.5	23.8	12.45	331.2	24.90
	1.00	c							
juice, light, no pulp	100.0	g		21	0.2	5.4	4.00	188.0	4.00
	240.0	g		50	0.5	13.0	9.60	451.2	9.60
	8.00	fl oz							
Mandarin, canned in light syrup	100.0	g		61	0.5	16.2	6.00	78.00	10.00
	252.0	g		154	1.1	40.8	15.12	196.6	25.20
	1.00	c							

LEMON	SERVING QUANTITY	SERVING UNIT	CALORIES (kCal)	PROTEIN (g)	TOTAL CARBOHYDRATES (g)	SODIUM (mg)	POTASSIUM (mg)	PHOSPHORUS (mg)	TOTAL FAT (g)
whole, without seeds	100.0	g	20	1.2	10.7	3.00	145.0	15.00	0.30
	108.0	g	22	1.3	11.6	3.24	156.6	16.20	0.32
	1.00	pc/ item							
peeled, 2-1/8" in diameter)	100.0	g	29	1.1	9.3	2.00	138.0	16.00	0.30
	58.00	g	17	0.6	5.4	1.16	80.04	9.28	0.17
	1.00	pc/ item							
juice, fresh	100.0	g	22	0.4	6.9	1.00	103.0	8.00	0.24
	30.50	g	7	0.1	2.1	0.31	31.42	2.44	0.07
	1.00	fl oz							
peel or zest	100.0	g	47	1.5	16.0	6.00	160.0	12.00	0.30
	2.00	g	1	0.0	0.3	0.12	3.20	0.24	0.01
	1.00	tsp							
pudding mix 1 svg = ½ c 1 package = 85g	100.0	g	363	0.1	91.8	506.0	5.00	3.00	0.50
	21.20	g	77	0.0	19.5	107.2	1.06	0.64	0.11
	1.00	svg							
juice, canned	100.0	g	17	0.5	5.6	24.00	109.0	9.00	0.07
	30.50	g	5	0.1	1.7	7.32	33.25	2.75	0.02
	1.00	fl oz							
soda, lemon lime	100.0	g	40	0.1	24.9	9.00	1.00	0.00	0.02
	245.6	g	98	0.1	10.1	22.10	2.46	0.00	0.05
	8.00	fl oz							
juice, unsweetened, frozen	100.0	g	22	0.5	6.5	1.00	89.00	8.00	0.32
	5.08	g	1	0.0	0.3	0.05	4.52	0.41	0.02
	1.00	tsp							
pudding, ready to eat 1 can= 5 oz	100.0	g	125	0.1	25.0	140.0	1.00	5.00	3.00
	142.0	g	178	0.1	35.5	198.8	1.42	7.10	4.26
	1.00	can/ item							
tea, black, sweetened, ready to drink	100.0	g	45	0.0	10.8	3.00	14.00	1.00	0.22
	271.0	g	122	0.0	29.3	8.13	37.94	2.71	0.60
	1.00	c							

LIME	SERVING QUANTITY	SERVING UNIT	CALORIES (kCal)	PROTEIN (g)	TOTAL CARBOHYDRATES (g)	SODIUM (mg)	POTASSIUM (mg)	PHOSPHORUS (mg)	TOTAL FAT (g)
whole, 2" in diameter	100.0	g	30	0.7	10.5	2.00	102.0	18.00	0.20
	67.00	g	20	0.5	7.1	1.34	68.34	12.06	0.13
	1.00	pc/ item							
juice, fresh	100.0	g	25	0.4	8.4	2.00	117.0	14.00	0.07
	5.13	g	1	0.0	0.4	0.10	6.01	0.72	0.00
	1.00	tsp							
juice, unsweetened, canned	100.0	g	21	0.3	6.7	16.00	75.00	10.00	0.23
	246.0	g	52	0.6	16.5	39.36	184.5	24.60	0.57
	1.00	c							
frozen ice dessert	100.0	g	128	0.4	32.6	22.00	3.00	1.00	0.00
	99.00	g	127	0.4	32.3	21.78	2.97	0.99	0.00
	0.50	c							
LYCHEE									
whole, fresh	100.0	g	66	0.8	16.5	1.00	171.0	31.00	0.44
	142.5	g	94	1.2	23.6	1.43	243.7	44.18	0.63
	0.75	c							
dried	100.0	g	277	3.8	70.7	3.00	1,110	181.00	1.20
	40.00	g	111	1.5	28.3	1.20	444.0	72.40	0.48
	16.00	pcs/ items							
MANGO									
whole, fresh	100.0	g	60	0.8	15.0	1.00	168.0	14.00	0.38
	207.0	g	124	1.7	31.0	2.07	347.8	28.98	0.79
	1.00	pc/ item							
dried, sweetened	100.0	g	319	2.5	78.6	162.00	279.0	50.00	1.18
nectar, canned	100.0	g	51	0.1	13.1	5.00	24.00	2.00	0.06
	251.0	g	128	0.3	32.9	12.55	60.24	5.02	0.15
	1.00	c							

APRICOT	SERVING QUANTITY	SERVING UNIT	CALORIES (kCal)	PROTEIN (g)	TOTAL CARBOHYDRATES (g)	SODIUM (mg)	POTASSIUM (mg)	PHOSPHORUS (mg)	TOTAL FAT (g)
whole, fresh	100.0	g	48	1.4	11.1	1.00	259.0	23.00	0.39
	140.0	g	67	2.0	15.6	1.40	362.6	32.20	0.55
	4.00	pcs/ items							
jam or preserves	100.0	g	242	0.7	64.4	40.00	77.00	3.00	0.20
1 packet = 0.5 oz = 14g	20.00	g	48	0.1	12.9	8.00	15.40	0.60	0.04
	1.00	tbsp							
nectar, canned	100.0	g	56	0.2	13.6	8.00	67.00	5.00	0.45
	251.0	g	141	0.4	34.2	20.08	168.2	12.55	1.13
	8.00	fl oz							
sweetened, frozen	100.0	g	98	0.7	25.1	4.00	229.0	19.00	0.10
	242.0	g	237	1.7	60.7	9.68	554.2	45.98	0.24
	1.00	c							
dehydrated, sulfured	100.0	g	320	4.9	82.9	13.00	1,850	157.0	0.62
	30.00	g	96	1.5	24.9	3.90	555.0	47.10	0.19
	0.25	c							
dried, halves, sulfured	100.0	g	241	3.4	62.6	10.00	1,162	71.00	0.51
	43.33	g	104	1.5	27.1	4.33	503.5	30.77	0.22
	0.33	c							
halves w/ skin, canned in juice	100.0	g	48	0.6	12.3	4.00	165.0	20.00	0.04
	244.0	g	117	1.5	30.1	9.76	402.6	48.80	0.10
	1.00	c							
halves with skin, canned in light syrup	100.0	g	63	0.5	16.5	4.00	138.0	32.89	0.05
	253.0	g	159	1.3	41.7	10.12	349.1	13.00	0.13
	1.00	c							
PLUM									
whole, fresh, sliced	100.0	g	46	0.7	11.4	0.00	157.0	16.00	0.28
	165.0	g	76	1.2	18.8	0.00	259.1	26.40	0.46
	1.00	c							
sauce	100.0	g	184	0.9	42.8	538.0	259.0	22.00	1.04
	19.00	g	35	0.2	8.1	102.2	49.21	4.18	0.20
	1.00	tbsp							
purple, pitted, *canned in water*	100.0	g	41	0.4	11.0	1.00	126.0	13.00	0.01
	249.0	g	102	1.0	27.5	2.49	313.7	32.37	0.02
	1.00	c							
purple, *canned in juice*	100.0	g	58	0.5	15.2	1.00	154.0	15.00	0.02
	252.0	g	146	1.3	38.2	2.52	388.1	37.80	0.05
	1.00	c							

	Serving Quantity	Serving Unit	Calories (kCal)	Protein (g)	Total Carbohydrates (g)	Sodium (mg)	Potassium (mg)	Phosphorus (mg)	Total Fat (g)
PRUNE									
puree	100.0	g	257	2.1	65.1	23.00	852.0	72.00	0.20
	28.35	g	73	0.6	18.5	6.52	241.5	20.41	0.06
	1.00	oz							
dried	100.0	g	240	2.2	63.9	2.00	732.0	69.00	0.38
	42.50	g	102	0.9	27.2	0.85	311.1	29.33	0.16
	0.25	c							
juice, canned	100.0	g	71	0.6	17.5	4.00	276.0	25.00	0.03
	256.0	g	182	1.6	44.7	10.24	706.5	64.00	0.08
	8.00	fl oz							
dehydrated, stewed	100.0	g	113	1.2	29.7	2.00	353.0	37.00	0.24
	36.40	g	41	0.5	10.8	0.73	128.5	13.47	0.09
	0.13	c							
dehydrated, low moisture	100.0	g	339	3.7	89.1	5.00	1,058	112.00	0.73
	33.00	g	112	1.2	29.4	1.65	349.1	36.96	0.24
	0.25	c							
RHUBARB									
whole, fresh, diced	100.0	g	21	0.9	4.5	4.00	288.0	14.00	0.20
	81.33	g	17	0.7	3.7	3.25	234.2	11.39	0.16
	0.67	c							
diced, frozen	100.0	g	21	0.6	5.1	2.00	108.0	12.00	0.11
	137.0	g	29	0.8	7.0	2.74	147.9	16.44	0.15
	1.00	c							
frozen, cooked with sugar	100.0	g	116	0.4	31.2	1.00	96.00	8.00	0.05
	120.0	g	139	0.5	37.4	1.20	115.2	9.60	0.06
	0.50	c							
POMEGRANATE									
whole, fresh, 4" in diameter	100.0	g	83	1.7	18.7	3.00	236.0	36.00	1.17
	282.0	g	234	4.7	52.7	8.46	665.5	101.52	3.30
	1.00	pc/ item							
juice, bottled	100.0	g	54	0.2	13.1	9.00	214.0	11.00	0.29
	251.2	g	136	0.4	33.0	22.61	537.5	27.63	0.73
	8.00	fl oz							

PAPAYA	SERVING QUANTITY	SERVING UNIT	CALORIES (kCal)	PROTEIN (g)	TOTAL CARBOHYDRATES (g)	SODIUM (mg)	POTASSIUM (mg)	PHOSPHORUS (mg)	TOTAL FAT (g)
whole, fresh, cubes	100.0	g	43	0.5	10.8	8.00	182.0	10.00	0.26
	140.0	g	60	0.7	15.2	11.20	254.8	14.00	0.36
	1.00	c							
nectar, canned	100.0	g	57	0.2	14.5	5.00	31.00	0.00	0.15
	250.0	g	143	0.4	36.3	12.50	77.50	0.00	0.38
	8.00	fl oz							
canned with heavy syrup, drained	100.0	g	206	0.1	55.8	9.00	67.00	6.00	0.55
	39.00	g	80	0.1	21.8	3.51	26.13	2.34	0.21
	1.00	pc/ chunk							
NECTARINE									
whole, fresh, slices	100.0	g	44	1.1	10.6	0.00	201.0	26.00	0.32
	138.0	g	61	1.5	14.7	0.00	277.3	35.88	0.44
	1.00	c							
PERSIMMON									
whole, fresh	100.0	g	127	0.8	33.5	1.00	310.0	26.00	0.40
	25.00	g	32	0.2	8.4	0.25	77.50	6.50	0.10
	1.00	pc/ item							
Japanese, fresh, 2-1/2" in diameter	100.0	g	70	0.6	18.6	1.00	161.0	17.00	0.19
	168.0	g	118	1.0	31.2	1.68	270.5	28.56	0.32
	1.00	pc/item							
Japanese, dried	100.0	g	274	1.4	73.4	2.00	802.0	81.00	0.59
	34.00	g	93	0.5	25.0	0.68	272.6	27.54	0.20
	1.00	pc/ item							
PURPLE PASSION FRUIT/ GRANADILLA									
whole, fresh - no refuse	100.0	g	97	2.2	23.4	28.00	348.0	68.00	0.70
	18.00	g	18	0.4	4.2	5.04	62.60	12.20	0.13
	1.00	pc/ fruit							
nectar, no ice	100.0	g	67	1.2	17.4	4.00	112.0	5.00	0.06
	31.00	g	21	0.1	5.4	1.24	34.70	1.55	0.02
	1.00	fl oz							
juice, purple passion fruit	100.0	g	51	0.4	13.6	6.00	278.0	13.00	0.05
	30.90	g	16	0.1	4.2	1.85	85.90	4.02	0.02
	1.00	fl oz							
juice, yellow passion fruit	100.0	g	60	0.7	14.5	6.00	278.0	25.00	0.18
	30.90	g	19	0.2	4.5	1.85	85.90	7.72	0.06
	1.00	fl oz							

WATER MELON

Food	Serving Quantity	Serving Unit	Calories (kCal)	Protein (g)	Total Carbohydrates (g)	Sodium (mg)	Potassium (mg)	Phosphorus (mg)	Total Fat (g)
raw, balls	100.0	g	30	0.6	7.6	1.00	112.0	11.00	0.15
	154.0	g	46	0.9	11.6	1.54	172.0	16.00	0.23
	1.00	c							
juice, 100%, no ice	100.0	g	30	0.6	7.6	1.00	112.0	11.00	0.15
	30.00	g	9	0.2	2.3	0.30	33.60	3.30	0.05
	1.00	fl oz							
seeds, kernels, dried	100.0	g	557	28.3	15.3	99.00	648.0	755.0	47.37
	28.35	g	158	8.0	4.3	28.10	184.0	214.0	13.40
	1.00	oz							

FIG

Food	Serving Quantity	Serving Unit	Calories (kCal)	Protein (g)	Total Carbohydrates (g)	Sodium (mg)	Potassium (mg)	Phosphorus (mg)	Total Fat (g)
raw	100.0	g	74	0.8	19.2	1.00	232.0	14.00	0.30
	50.00	g	37	0.4	9.6	0.50	116.0	7.00	0.15
	1.00	pc/ item							
dried	100.0	g	249	3.3	63.9	10.00	680.0	67.00	0.92
	8.00	g	20	0.3	5.1	0.80	54.40	5.36	0.07
	1.00	pc							
canned	100.0	g	75	0.6	19.4	1.00	157.0	10.00	0.24
	250.0	g	188	1.4	48.4	2.50	392.0	25.00	0.60
	1.00	c							
dried, stewed	100.0	g	107	1.4	27.6	4.00	294.0	29.00	0.40
	259.0	g	277	3.7	71.4	10.40	761.0	75.10	1.04
	1.00	c							
canned, water pack, solids/liquids	100.0	g	53	0.4	14.0	1.00	103.0	10.00	0.10
	248.0	g	131	1.0	34.7	2.48	255.0	24.80	0.25
	1.00	c							
canned, light syrup pack, solids/liquids	100.0	g	69	0.4	18.0	1.00	102.0	10.00	0.10
	252.0	g	174	1.0	45.2	2.52	257.0	25.20	0.25
	1.00	c							

GUAVA

Food	Serving Quantity	Serving Unit	Calories (kCal)	Protein (g)	Total Carbohydrates (g)	Sodium (mg)	Potassium (mg)	Phosphorus (mg)	Total Fat (g)
raw	100.0	g	68	2.6	14.3	2.00	417.0	40.00	0.95
	55.00	g	37	1.4	7.9	1.10	229.0	22.00	0.52
	1.00	pc/ item							
nectar no ice	100.0	g	48	0.3	13.3	6.00	33.00	3.00	0.07
	31.00	g	15	0.1	4.1	1.86	10.20	0.93	0.02
	1.00	fl oz							
paste	100.0	g	280	0.1	77.6	2.00	69.00	3.00	0.27
	20.00	g	56	0.0	14.5	0.40	13.80	0.60	0.05
	1.00	tbsp							

DATES	SERVING QUANTITY	SERVING UNIT	CALORIES (kCal)	PROTEIN (g)	TOTAL CARBOHYDRATES (g)	SODIUM (mg)	POTASSIUM (mg)	PHOSPHORUS (mg)	TOTAL FAT (g)
whole, dried	100.0	g	282	2.5	75.0	2.00	656.0	62.00	0.39
	8.00	g	23	0.2	6.0	0.16	52.50	4.96	0.03
	1.00	pc/ item							
Medjool, pitted	100.0	g	277	1.8	75.0	1.00	696.0	62.00	0.15
	24.00	g	67	0.4	18.0	0.24	167.0	14.90	0.04
	1.00	pc/item							
candy	100.0	g	379	4.2	58.1	22.00	540.0	117.0	18.04
	28.35	g	107	1.2	16.5	6.24	153.0	33.20	5.11
	1.00	oz							
POMELO									
whole, fresh	100.0	g	38	0.8	9.6	1.00	216.0	17.00	0.04
section	190.0	g	72	1.4	18.3	1.90	410.0	32.30	0.08
	1.00	c							
MANGOSTEEN									
canned, syrup pack	100.0	g	73	0.4	17.9	7.00	48.00	8.00	0.58
drained	196.0	g	143	0.8	35.1	13.70	94.10	15.70	1.14
	1.00	c							
JACKFRUIT									
raw, fresh	100.0	g	95	1.7	23.3	2.00	448.0	21.00	0.64
slices	165.0	g	157	2.8	38.4	3.30	739.0	34.60	1.06
	1.00	c							
canned, syrup pack	100.0	g	92	0.4	23.9	11.00	96.00	6.00	0.14
drained	178.0	g	164	0.6	42.6	19.60	171.0	10.70	0.25
	1.00	c							
DURIAN									
raw or frozen	100.0	g	147	1.5	27.1	2.00	436.0	39.00	5.33
chopped or diced	243.0	g	357	3.6	65.8	4.86	1,060	94.80	13.00
	1.00	c							
SOURSOP									
raw, pulp	100.0	g	66	1.0	16.8	14.00	278.0	27.00	0.30
	225.0	g	148	2.3	37.9	31.50	626.0	60.80	0.68
	1.00	c							
nectar	100.0	g	59	0.1	14.9	8.00	25.00	2.00	0.17
no ice, pure	31.00	g	18	0.0	4.6	2.48	7.75	0.62	0.05
	1.00	fl oz							

PLANTAIN	SERVING QUANTITY	SERVING UNIT	CALORIES (KCal)	PROTEIN (g)	TOTAL CARBOHYDRATES (g)	SODIUM (mg)	POTASSIUM (mg)	PHOSPHORUS (mg)	TOTAL FAT (g)
ripe, raw, fresh	100.0	g	122	1.3	31.9	4.00	487.0	32.00	0.35
	180.0	g	220	2.3	57.4	7.20	877.0	57.60	0.63
	1.00	pc/ item							
green, raw, fresh	100.0	g	152	1.3	36.7	2.00	431.0	31.00	0.07
	267.0	g	406	3.3	97.9	5.34	1,150	82.80	0.19
	1.00	pc/item							
green, boiled	100.0	g	121	1.1	29.2	2.00	289.0	24.00	0.08
	137.0	g	166	1.5	39.9	2.74	396.0	32.90	0.11
	1.00	c							
green, fried	100.0	g	309	1.5	49.2	2.00	482.0	44.00	11.81
	118.0	g	365	1.8	58.0	2.36	569.0	51.90	13.90
	1.00	c							
yellow, raw, fresh	100.0	g	122	1.3	31.9	4.00	487.0	32.00	0.35
	270.0	g	329	3.5	86.1	10.8	1,310	86.40	0.95
	1.00	pc/ item							
yellow, baked	100.0	g	155	1.5	41.4	2.00	477.0	37.00	0.16
	139.0	g	215	2.1	57.5	2.78	663.0	51.40	0.22
	1.00	c							
chips	100.0	g	531	2.3	63.8	202	786.0	78.00	29.59
	28.35	g	151	0.6	18.1	57.3	223.0	22.10	8.39
	1.00	oz							

AVOCADO	SERVING QUANTITY	SERVING UNIT	CALORIES (KCal)	PROTEIN (g)	TOTAL CARBOHYDRATES (g)	SODIUM (mg)	POTASSIUM (mg)	PHOSPHORUS (mg)	TOTAL FAT (g)
fresh, raw	100.0	g	160	2.0	8.5	7.00	485.0	52.00	14.66
mashed/ pureed	230.0	g	368	4.6	19.6	16.1	1,120	120.0	33.70
	1.00	c							
oil	100.0	g	884	0.0	0.0	0.00	0.00	0.00	100.0
	14.00	g	124	0.0	0.0	0.00	0.00	0.00	14.00
	1.00	tbsp							
dressing	100.0	g	427	1.9	7.4	867	58.00	31.00	43.33
	15.30	g	65	0.3	1.1	133.	8.87	4.74	6.63
	1.00	tbsp							
California, raw/fresh	100.0	g	167	2.0	8.6	8.00	507.0	54.00	15.41
no seed and skin	136.0	g	227	2.7	11.8	10.9	690.0	73.40	21.00
	1.00	pc/ item							
Florida, fresh/ raw	100.0	g	120	2.2	7.8	2.00	351.0	40.00	10.06
no seed and skin	304.0	g	365	6.8	23.8	6.08	1,070	122.0	30.60
	1.00	pc/ item							
Guacamole	100.0	g	155	2.0	8.5	344	472.0	51.00	14.18
	15.00	g	23	0.3	1.3	51.6	70.80	7.65	2.13
	1.00	tbsp							

TAMARIND	SERVING QUANTITY	SERVING UNIT	CALORIES (kCal)	PROTEIN (g)	TOTAL CARBOHYDRATES (g)	SODIUM (mg)	POTASSIUM (mg)	PHOSPHORUS (mg)	TOTAL FAT (g)
fresh, raw	100.0	g	239	2.8	62.5	28.00	628	113	0.60
	2.00	g	5	0.1	1.3	0.56	12.60	2.26	0.01
	1.00	pc/item							
candy	100.0	g	331	0.0	92.0	1,643	309.0	56.00	0.00
	22.00	g	73	0.0	20.2	361.0	68.00	12.30	0.00
	1.00	tbsp							
dried	100.0	g	254	2.5	66.2	25.00	565	102	0.57
	160.0	g	406	4.0	106	40.00	904	163	0.91
	1.00	c							
SAPODILLA									
fresh/raw	100.0	g	83	0.4	20.0	12.00	193	12.00	1.10
	170.0	g	141	0.8	33.9	20.40	328	20.40	1.87
	1.00	pc/ item							
SUGARAPPLE *(Sweetsop)*									
fresh, raw	100.0	g	94	2.1	23.6	9.00	247	32.00	0.29
(2-7/8" in diameter)	155.0	g	146	3.2	36.6	14.00	383	49.60	0.45
	1.00	pc/ item							
STARFRUIT									
fresh/ raw	100.0	g	31	1.0	6.7	2.00	133	12.00	0.33
	90.00	g	28	0.9	6.1	1.80	120.0	10.80	0.30
	1.00	pc/ item							

D. Carbohydrates

(Grains, Breads, Pasta/Noodles, Cereals)

Hey there!

Do you need to print out this Food List?

You can download a printable version of this chart by scanning the QR code below or copying the link on your computer browser.

https://go.renaltracker.com/printfoodlist

BREADS	SERVING QUANTITY	SERVING UNIT	CALORIES (kCal)	PROTEIN (g)	TOTAL CARBOHYDRATES (g)	SODIUM (mg)	POTASSIUM (mg)	PHOSPHORUS (mg)	TOTAL FAT (g)
whole wheat	100.0	g	252	12.5	42.7	455.0	254	212.0	3.50
	50.00	g	126	6.2	21.4	227.5	127.0	106.0	1.75
	2.00	slices							
white	100.0	g	266	8.9	49.4	490.0	126.0	98.00	490.0
	50.00	g	133	4.4	24.7	245.0	63.00	49.00	245.0
	2.00	slices							
french, small (2'x2.5'x1.75')	100.0	g	272	10.8	51.9	602.0	117.0	105.0	2.42
	32.00	g	87	3.4	16.6	192.6	37.44	33.60	0.77
	1.00	slice							
pita, 6.5"	100.0	g	275	9.1	55.7	536.0	120.0	97.00	1.20
	60.00	g	165	5.5	33.4	321.6	72.00	58.20	0.72
	1.00	pc							
sourdough	100.0	g	272	10.8	51.9	602.0	117.0	105.0	2.42
	50.00	g	136	5.4	25.9	301.0	58.50	52.50	1.21
	2.00	slices							
rye	100.0	g	259	8.5	48.3	603.0	166.0	125.0	33.00
	32.00	g	83	2.7	15.5	192.9	53.12	40.00	1.06
	1.00	slice							
bagels, wheat	100.0	g	250	10.2	48.9	439.0	165.0	142.0	1.53
	105.0	g	262	10.7	51.3	461.0	173.0	149.0	1.61
	1.00	reg pc							
biscuits	100.0	g	362	7.5	43.9	930.0	184.0	501.0	18.19
	45.00	g	163	3.4	19.8	418.0	82.80	225.0	8.19
	1.00	pc							
sprouted, wheat	100.0	g	188	13.2	33.9	474.0	198.0	176.0	0.00
	26.00	g	49	3.4	8.8	123.0	51.50	45.80	0.00
	1.00	slice							
cracked, wheat	100.0	g	274	10.7	47.5	473.0	141.0	129.0	4.53
	28.00	g	77	3.0	13.3	132.0	39.50	36.10	1.27
	1.00	reg slice							
tortillas, corn	100.0	g	218	5.7	44.6	45.00	186.0	314.0	2.85
ready-to-bake or fry	24.00	g	52	1.4	10.7	10.80	44.60	75.40	0.68
	1.00	Pc							
tortillas, flour	100.0	g	306	8.2	49.4	736.0	125.0	206.0	7.99
approx. 6" diameter	30.00	g	92	2.5	14.8	221.0	37.50	61.80	2.40
ready-to-bake or fry, refrigerated	1.00	pc							

BREADS	SERVING QUANTITY	SERVING UNIT	CALORIES (kCal)	PROTEIN (g)	TOTAL CARBOHYDRATES (g)	SODIUM (mg)	POTASSIUM (mg)	PHOSPHORUS (mg)	TOTAL FAT (g)
tortilla, whole wheat	100.0	g	310	9.8	45.9	617.0	262.0	346.0	9.76
ready-to-bake or fry	41.00	g	127	4.0	18.8	253.0	107.0	142.0	4.00
	1.00	pc							
ciabatta	100.0	g	259	9.5	48.1	618.0	124.0	95.00	2.73
(yeast bread)	43.00	g	111	4.1	20.7	266.0	53.30	40.80	1.17
Italian, Grecian, Armenian thick sllice	1.00	pc							
focaccia, plain	100.0	g	249	8.8	35.8	561.0	114.0	128.0	7.89
(Italian flatbread)	57.00	g	142	5.0	20.4	320.0	65.00	73.00	4.50
	1.00	pc							
Pita, medium	100.0	g	275	9.1	55.7	536.0	120.0	97.00	1.20
	57.00	g	157	5.2	31.7	306.0	68.40	55.30	0.68
	1.00	pc							
Naan, *plain*	100.0	g	291	9.6	50.4	465.0	125.0	100.0	5.65
	90.00	g	262	8.7	45.4	418.0	112.0	90.00	5.08
	1.00	pc							
Paratha, whole	100.0	g	326	6.4	45.4	467.0	185.0	188.0	6.70
wheat, frozen	79.00	g	258	5.0	35.9	495.0	196.0	199.0	7.10
	1.00	pc							
brioche	100.0	g	418	8.8	35.8	452.0	139.0	120.0	13.20
	77.00	g	322	6.7	27.6	357.0	110.0	94.80	10.40
	1.00	pc							
croissants, plain	100.0	g	406	8.2	45.8	440.0	120.0	125.0	26.80
medium	57.00	g	231	4.7	26.1	339.0	92.40	96.20	20.60
	1.00	pc							
croissants, chocolate	100.0	g	421	7.4	49.4	384.0	118.0	105.0	21.00
	57.00	g	240	4.2	28.2	219.0	67.30	59.80	12.00
	1.00	pc							
croissants, cheese	100.0	g	414	9.2	47.0	361.0	132.0	130.0	20.90
	57.00	g	236	5.2	26.8	206.0	75.22	74.10	11.90
	1.00	pc							
muffins,	100.0	g	245	7.0	50.2	386.0	130.0	127.0	1.75
english, whole	57.00	g	140	4.0	28.6	220.0	74.10	72.40	1.00
grain white	1.00	pc							
muffins,	100.0	g	203	8.8	40.4	364.0	210.0	282.0	2.10
english,	66.00	g	134	5.8	26.7	240.0	139.0	186.0	1.39
whole wheat	1.00	pc							

BREADS

BREADS	SERVING QUANTITY	SERVING UNIT	CALORIES (kCal)	PROTEIN (g)	TOTAL CARBOHYDRATES (g)	SODIUM (mg)	POTASSIUM (mg)	PHOSPHORUS (mg)	TOTAL FAT (g)
muffins, english, *mixed-grain includes granola*	100.0	g	235	9.1	46.3	298.0	156.0	81.00	1.80
	66.00	g	155	6.0	30.6	197.0	103.0	53.40	1.19
	1.00	pc							
pumpernickle, med or regular slice	100.0	g	250	8.7	47.5	596.0	208.0	178.0	3.10
	32.00	g	80	2.8	15.2	191.0	66.60	57.00	0.99
	1.00	pc							
cinammon, medium or regular slice	100.0	g	253	7.1	44.4	388.0	74.00	57.00	5.29
	28.00	g	71	2.0	12.4	109.0	20.70	16.00	1.48
	1.00	pc							
raisin, med or regular slice	100.0	g	273	8.8	52.2	432.0	180.0	112.0	3.26
	28.00	g	76	2.5	14.6	121.0	50.40	31.40	0.91
	1.00	pc							
roll, multigrain med, reg, sandwich size	100.0	g	263	9.6	44.6	458.0	160.0	122.0	6.00
	43.00	g	113	4.1	19.2	197.0	68.80	52.50	2.58
	1.00	pc							
bread stuffing, homemade	100.0	g	177	3.1	21.7	471.0	72.00	41.00	8.51
dry mix, prepared	228.0	g	404	7.2	49.5	1,070	164.0	93.50	19.40
	1.00	pc							

GRITS

GRITS	SERVING QUANTITY	SERVING UNIT	CALORIES (kCal)	PROTEIN (g)	TOTAL CARBOHYDRATES (g)	SODIUM (mg)	POTASSIUM (mg)	PHOSPHORUS (mg)	TOTAL FAT (g)
corn, yellow, quick,	100.0	g	59	1.4	12.9	2.00	21.00	11.00	0.19
	242.0	g	143	3.4	31.2	4.84	50.82	26.62	0.46
unenriched cooked with water, no salt	1.00	c							
corn, white, quick,	100.0	g	59	1.4	12.9	2.00	21.00	11.00	0.19
	242.0	g	143	3.4	31.2	4.84	50.82	26.62	0.46
unenriched cooked with water	1.00	c							
POLENTA	100.0	g							
(cornmeal)	240.0	g	139	2.7	30.	170.0	50.40	36.00	0.67
	1	c							

PASTA

PASTA	SERVING QUANTITY	SERVING UNIT	CALORIES (KCal)	PROTEIN (g)	TOTAL CARBOHYDRATES (g)	SODIUM (mg)	POTASSIUM (mg)	PHOSPHORUS (mg)	TOTAL FAT (g)
spaghetti, unenriched, cooked	100.0	g	158	5.8	30.9	1.00	44.00	58.00	0.93
	70.00	g	111	4.1	21.6	0.70	30.80	40.60	0.65
	0.50	c							
spaghetti, enriched, cooked	100.0	g	158	5.8	30.9	1.00	44.00	58.00	0.93
	140.0	g	221	8.1	43.2	1.40	61.60	81.20	1.30
	1.00	c							
spaghetti, whole wheat, cooked	100.0	g	149	6.0	30.1	4.00	96.00	127.0	1.71
	140.0	g	209	8.4	42.1	5.60	134.4	177.8	2.39
	1.00	c							
bowtie/farfalle, enriched, cooked	100.0	g	136	4.8	27.4	1.10	24.51	-na-	0.55
	154.8	g	210	7.4	42.3	0.16	37.93	-na-	0.86
	1.00	c							
fusilli, enriched, cooked	100.0	g	161	5.7	32.5	1.30	29.09	-na-	0.66
	130.4	g	210	7.4	42.3	1.70	37.93	-na-	0.86
	1.00	c							
penne, enriched, cooked	100.0	g	169	6.0	34.1	1.37	30.55	-na-	0.69
	124.1	g	210	7.4	42.3	1.70	37.93	-na-	0.86
	1.00	c							
macaroni, enriched, cooked	100.0	g	133	4.7	26.8	1.08	24.04	-na-	0.54
	157.8	g	210	7.4	42.3	1.70	37.93	-na-	0.86
	1.00	c							
lasagna, enriched, boiled/drained	100.0	g	150	5.3	30.1	1.21	26.98	-na-	0.61
	140.6	g	210	7.4	42.3	1.70	37.93	-na-	0.86
	1.00	c							
whole grain, 51%whole wheat rest enriched semolina, cooked spaghetti, unenriched, cooked	100.0	g	156	5.7	30.9	4.00	71.00	97.00	1.48

CRACKERS	SERVING QUANTITY	SERVING UNIT	CALORIES (KCal)	PROTEIN (g)	TOTAL CARBOHYDRATES (g)	SODIUM (mg)	POTASSIUM (mg)	PHOSPHORUS (mg)	TOTAL FAT (g)
melba toast, rye	100.0	g	389	11.6	77.3	899.0	193.0	183.0	3.40
3 3/4" x 1 3/4" x 1/8"	15.00	g	58	1.7	11.6	134.8	28.95	27.45	0.51
	3.00	pcs							
melba toast, wheat	100.0	g	374	12.9	76.4	837.0	148.0	165.0	2.30
	15.00	g	56	1.9	11.5	125.5	22.20	24.75	0.35
	3.00	pcs							
saltine, low salt (square)	100.0	g	421	9.5	74.3	198.0	724.0	111.0	8.85
	15.00	g	63	1.4	11.2	29.70	108.6	16.65	1.33
	5.00	pcs							
saltine, fat-free, low sodium	100.0	g	393	10.5	82.3	849.0	115.0	113.0	1.60
	15.00	g	59	1.6	12.4	127.3	17.25	16.95	0.24
	3.00	pcs							
saltines, whole wheat/multi-grain	100.0	g	398	7.1	68.3	1,214	221.0	196.0	10.71
	14.00	g	56	1.0	9.6	169.9	30.94	27.44	1.50
	1.00	svg							
whole wheat, low salt	100.0	g	443	8.8	68.6	186.0	297.0	295.0	17.20
	28.00	g	124	2.5	19.2	52.08	83.16	82.60	4.82
	7.00	pcs							
whole wheat, reduced fat	100.0	g	416	11.3	75.5	745.0	373.0	364.0	7.59
1 svg= 29g	4.20	g	17	0.5	3.2	31.29	15.67	15.29	0.32
	1.00	pcs							
graham, plain or honey, low fat	100.0	g	386	5.7	78.0	629.0	171.0	163.0	5.71
	35.00	g	135	2.0	27.3	220.1	59.85	57.05	2.00
	1.00	svg							
goldfish (fish-shaped), flavored	100.0	g	463	10.2	65.7	970.0	224.0	167.0	17.71
	5.20	g	24	0.5	3.4	50.44	11.65	8.68	0.92
	10.00	pcs							
toast thins, low sodium	100.0	g	442	6.5	67.7	177.0	306.0	266.0	16.13
	31.00	g	137	2.0	21.0	54.87	94.86	82.46	5.00
	1.00	svg							

RICE

RICE	SERVING QUANTITY	SERVING UNIT	CALORIES (kCal)	PROTEIN (g)	TOTAL CARBOHYDRATES (g)	SODIUM (mg)	POTASSIUM (mg)	PHOSPHORUS (mg)	TOTAL FAT (g)
white, unenriched	100.0	g	359	6.9	79.8	5.00	75.00	94.00	1.30
white, cooked, glutinous	100.0	g	96	2.0	21.0	5.00	20.00	33.00	0.27
	174.0	g	167	3.5	36.5	6.60	26.40	43.60	0.36
	1.00	c							
white, long-grain, parboiled enriched, cooked	100.0	g	123	2.9	26.1	0.00	29.00	37.00	0.21
	158.0	g	194	4.6	41.2	0.00	53.90	68.80	0.39
	1.00	c							
flour, white, unenriched	100.0	g	359	6.9	79.8	0.00	26.00	33.00	0.19
white, steamed, Chinese restaurant cup, loosely packed	100.0	g	151	3.2	33.9	0.00	53.30	67.60	0.39
	132.0	g	199	4.2	44.7	1.00	265.0	319.0	3.85
	1.00	c							
white, medium-grain, cooked unenriched	100.0	g	130	2.4	28.6	201.0	86.00	102.0	0.96
	186.0	g	242	4.4	53.2	394.0	169.0	200.0	1.88
	1.00	c							
white, short-grain, cooked unenriched	100.0	g	130	2.4	28.7	3.00	101.0	82.00	0.34
	205.0	g	266	4.8	58.8	4.92	166.0	134.0	0.56
	1.00	c							
flour, brown,	100.0	g	365	7.2	75.5	7.00	427.0	433.0	1.08
brown, cooked, no salt, no fat	100.0	g	122	2.7	25.5	11.20	683.0	693.0	1.73
	196.0	g	239	5.4	49.9	5.00	75.00	94.00	1.30
	1.00	c							
wild, cooked	100.0	g	101	4.0	21.3	5.00	20.00	33.00	0.27
	164.0	g	166	6.5	35.0	6.60	26.40	43.60	0.36
	1.00	c							
wild, raw	100.0	g	357	14.7	74.9	0.00	29.00	37.00	0.21
	160.0	g	571	23.6	120	0.00	53.90	68.80	0.39
	1.00	c							

OATS

OATS	SERVING QUANTITY	SERVING UNIT	CALORIES (kCal)	PROTEIN (g)	TOTAL CARBOHYDRATES (g)	SODIUM (mg)	POTASSIUM (mg)	PHOSPHORUS (mg)	TOTAL FAT (g)
raw	100.0	g	379	12.2	67.7	6.00	362.0	410.0	6.52
	81.00	g	307	10.7	54.8	4.86	293.0	332.0	5.28
	1.00	c							
cereal, oat,	100.0	g	372	12.4	73.2	497.0	633.0	357.0	6.60
	33.00	g	123	4.1	24.2	164.0	209.0	118.0	2.18
	1.00	c							
steel cut	100.0	g	378	13.3	66.7	0.00	356.0	na	6.67
Brand: ARROWHEAD MILLS	45.00	g	170	6.0	30.0	0.00	160.0	na	3.00
	1.00	svg							
rolled	100.0	g	350	12.5	67.5	0.00	350.0	na	6.25
Brand: MILLVILLE by Aldi	40.00	g	140	5.0	27.0	0.00	140.0	na	2.50
	1.00	svg							
bran, cooked	100.0	g	40	3.2	11.4	1.00	92.00	119.0	0.86
	219.0	g	88	7.0	25.1	2.19	201.0	261.0	1.88
	1.00	c							
bran, uncooked (raw)	100.0	g	246	17.3	66.2	4.00	566.0	734.0	7.03
	94.00	g	231	16.3	62.2	3.76	532.0	690.0	6.61
	1.00	c							
flour, partially debranned	100.0	g	404	14.7	65.7	19.00	371.0	452.0	9.12
	104.0	g	420	15.2	68.3	19.80	386.0	470.0	9.48
	1.00	c							
regular, rolled, not fortified, dry	100.0	g	379	13.2	67.7	6.00	362.0	410.0	6.52
	81.00	g	307	10.7	54.8	4.86	293.0	332.0	5.28
	1.00	c							

WHEAT	SERVING QUANTITY	SERVING UNIT	CALORIES (kCal)	PROTEIN (g)	TOTAL CARBOHYDRATES (g)	SODIUM (mg)	POTASSIUM (mg)	PHOSPHORUS (mg)	TOTAL FAT (g)
durum	100.0	g	399	13.7	71.1	2.00	431.0	508.0	2.47
	192.0	g	651	26.3	137	3.84	828.0	975.0	4.74
	1.00	c							
sprouted	100.0	g	198	7.5	42.5	16.00	169.0	200.0	1.27
	108.0	g	214	8.1	45.9	17.30	183.0	216.0	1.37
	1.00	c							
germ	100.0	g	360	23.2	51.8	12.00	892.0	842.0	9.72
	115.0	g	414	26.7	59.6	13.80	1,030	968	11.20
	1.00	c							
bran	100.0	g	216	15.6	64.5	2.00	1,180	1,010	4.25
	58.00	g	125	9.1	37.4	1.16	684.0	586.0	2.46
	1.00	c							
cream of wheat, instant, dry	100.0	g	366	10.6	75.5	571.0	115.0	103.0	1.40
	11.50	g	42	1.2	8.7	65.70	13.20	11.80	0.16
	1.00	tbsp							
flour, whole wheat, unenriched	100.0	g	370	15.1	71.2	3.00	376.0	352.0	2.73
whole grain, soft wheat	100.0	g	332	9.6	74.5	3.00	394.0	323.0	1.95
bread flour, unenriched unsifted	100.0	g	361	12.0	72.5	2.00	100.0	97.00	1.66
	137.0	g	495	16.4	99.4	2.74	137.0	133.0	2.27
	1.00	c							
flour, bread, white, enriched	100.0	g	361	12.0	72.5	2.00	100.0	97.00	1.66
	137.0	g	495	16.4	99.4	2.74	137.0	133.0	2.27
	1.00	c							
flour, cake, enriched unsifted	100.0	g	362	8.2	78.0	2.00	105.0	85.00	0.86
	137.0	g	496	11.2	107	2.74	144.0	116.0	1.18
	1.00	c							

CUOSCUOS

	SERVING QUANTITY	SERVING UNIT	CALORIES (kCal)	PROTEIN (g)	TOTAL CARBOHYDRATES (g)	SODIUM (mg)	POTASSIUM (mg)	PHOSPHORUS (mg)	TOTAL FAT (g)
dry	100.0	g	376	12.8	77.4	10.00	166.0	170.0	0.64
	173.0	g	680	22.1	134	17.30	287.0	294.0	1.11
	1.00	c							
cooked	100.0	g	112	3.8	23.2	5.00	58.00	22.00	0.16
	157.0	g	176	6.0	36.4	7.85	91.10	34.50	0.25
	1.00	c							

BARLEY

	SERVING QUANTITY	SERVING UNIT	CALORIES (kCal)	PROTEIN (g)	TOTAL CARBOHYDRATES (g)	SODIUM (mg)	POTASSIUM (mg)	PHOSPHORUS (mg)	TOTAL FAT (g)
pearled, cooked	100.0	g	123	2.3	28.2	3.00	93.00	54.00	0.44
	157.0	g	193	3.6	44.3	4.71	146.0	84.80	0.69
	1.00	c							
flour or meal	100.0	g	345	10.5	74.5	4.00	309.0	296.0	1.60
	148.0	g	511	15.5	110.	5.92	457.0	438.0	2.37
	1.00	c							

QUINOA

	SERVING QUANTITY	SERVING UNIT	CALORIES (kCal)	PROTEIN (g)	TOTAL CARBOHYDRATES (g)	SODIUM (mg)	POTASSIUM (mg)	PHOSPHORUS (mg)	TOTAL FAT (g)
cooked	100.0	g	120	4.4	21.3	7.00	172.0	152.0	1.92
	185.0	g	222	8.1	39.4	13.00	318.0	281.0	3.55
	1.00	c							
uncooked	100.0	g	368	14.1	64.2	5.00	563.0	457.0	6.07
	170.0	g	626	24.0	109	8.50	957.0	777.0	10.30
	1.00	c							
pasta from quinoa flour	100.0	g	152	3.2	31.1	4.00	63.00	91.00	2.07
(gluten-free)	132.0	g	201	4.3	41.1	5.28	83.20	120.0	2.73
not packed	1.00	c							

AMARANTH

Grain	100.0	g	102	3.8	18.7	6.00	135.0	148.0	1.58
cooked	246.0	g	251	9.4	46.0	14.80	332.0	364.0	3.89
	1.00	c							

CEREALS

	SERVING QUANTITY	SERVING UNIT	CALORIES (kCal)	PROTEIN (g)	TOTAL CARBOHYDRATES (g)	SODIUM (mg)	POTASSIUM (mg)	PHOSPHORUS (mg)	TOTAL FAT (g)
corn flakes, plain (store brands)	100.0	g	357	7.5	84.1	729.0	168.0	102.0	0.40
	25.00	g	89	1.9	21.0	182.0	42.00	25.50	0.10
	1.00	c							
corn flakes, frosted (store brands)	100.0	g	389	4.3	90.2	451.0	82.00	46.00	0.87
	40.00	g	156	1.7	36.1	180.0	32.80	18.40	0.35
	1.00	c							
crispy rice	100.0	g	383	6.7	86.2	545.0	106.0	98.00	1.26
	26.00	g	100	1.7	22.4	142.0	27.60	25.50	0.33
	1.00	c							
cocoa puffs (General Mills)	100.0	g	383	5.6	83.7	564.0	272.0	222.0	5.20
	36.00	g	138	2.0	30.1	203.0	97.90	79.90	1.87
	1.00	c							
muesli, with fruits & nuts	100.0	g	335	8.6	74.9	239.0	324.0	225.0	5.40
	85.00	g	302	7.3	63.7	203.0	275.0	191.0	4.59
	1.00	c							
muesli Brand: Safeway	100.0	g	386	8.8	73.7	228.0	474.0	175.0	5.26
	57.00	g	220	5.0	42.0	130.0	270.0	99.80	3.00
	1.00	svg							
granola, homemade, ready-to-eat	100.0	g	489	13.7	53.9	26.00	539.0	431.0	24.30
	122.0	g	597	16.7	65.8	31.70	658.0	526.0	29.60
	1.00	c							
granola bars, plain	100.0	g	471	10.1	64.4	294.0	336.0	277.0	19.80
	28.00	g	132	2.8	18.0	82.30	94.10	77.60	5.54
	1.00	bar/ oz							
granola bars, almond	100.0	g	495	7.7	62.0	256.0	273.0	228.0	25.50
	28.35	g	140	2.2	17.6	72.60	77.40	64.60	7.23
	1.00	oz							

PANCAKE	SERVING QUANTITY	SERVING UNIT	CALORIES (kCal)	PROTEIN (g)	TOTAL CARBOHYDRATES (g)	SODIUM (mg)	POTASSIUM (mg)	PHOSPHORUS (mg)	TOTAL FAT (g)
buttermilk (from recipe)	100.0	g	227	6.8	28.7	522.0	145.0	139.0	9.30
	38.00	g	86	2.6	10.9	198.0	55.10	52.80	3.53
	1- 4" diameter	pc							
plain, (prepared from recipe)	100.0	g	227	6.4	28.3	439.0	132.0	159.0	9.70
	38.00	g	86	2.4	10.8	167.0	50.20	60.40	3.69
	1- 4" diameter	pc							
plain, reduced fat	100.0	g	269	5.7	57.3	429.0	97.00	190.0	1.90
	105.0	g	282	6.0	60.2	450.0	102.0	200.0	2.00
	3.00	pcs							
plain, frozen, ready to heat includes buttermilk	100.0	g	233	5.2	37.8	461.0	90.00	215.0	6.83
	40.00	g	93	2.1	15.1	184.0	36.00	86.00	2.73
	1 (4")	pc							
gluten-free, frozen, ready to heat	100.0	g	215	3.3	40.3	331.0	127.0	306.0	4.55
	48.00	g	103	1.6	19.3	159.0	61.00	147.0	2.18
	1.00	pc							
WAFFLE									
plain, prepared from recipe	100.0	g	291	7.9	32.9	511.0	159.0	190.0	14.10
	75.00	g	218	5.9	24.7	383.0	119.0	142.0	10.60
	1 (7")	pc							

E. Milk and Cheeses

(Dairy and Non-Dairy)

Hey there!

Do you need to print out this Food List?

You can download a printable version of this chart by scanning the QR code below or copying the link on your computer browser.

https://go.renaltracker.com/printfoodlist

MILK

	SERVING QUANTITY	SERVING UNIT	CALORIES (kCal)	PROTEIN (g)	TOTAL CARBOHYDRATES (g)	SODIUM (mg)	POTASSIUM (mg)	PHOSPHORUS (mg)	TOTAL FAT (g)
(cow) whole	100.0	g	60	3.3	4.7	38.0	150.0	101.0	3.20
	244.0	g	146	8.0	11.4	92.7	366.0	246.0	7.81
	1	c							
2% reduced fat	100.0	g	50	3.4	4.9	39.0	159.0	103.0	1.90
	244.0	g	122	8.2	12.0	95.2	388.0	251.0	4.64
	1	c							
low fat (1%)	100.0	g	43	3.4	5.2	39.0	159.0	103.0	0.95
	244.0	g	105	8.3	12.7	95.2	388.0	251.0	2.32
	1	c							
skim, fat free	100.0	g	34	3.4	4.9	41.0	167.0	107.0	0.08
	244.0	g	83	8.4	11.9	100.0	407.0	261.0	0.20
	1	c							
lactose free, from whole milk	100.0	g	60	3.3	4.7	38.0	150.0	101.0	3.20
	244.0	g	146	8.0	11.4	92.7	366.0	246.0	7.81
	1	c							
Buttermilk, dried	100.0	g	387	34.3	49.0	517.0	1592	933	5.78
	6.5	g	25	2.2	3.2	33.6	103.0	60.60	0.38
	1	tbsp							
buttermilk, fluid, whole	100.0	g	62	3.2	4.9	105.0	135.0	85.00	3.31
	245.0	g	152	7.9	12.0	257.0	331.0	208.0	8.11
	1	c							
condensed, sweetened	100.0	g	321	7.9	54.4	127.0	371.0	253.0	8.70
	38.0	g	122	3.0	20.7	48.3	141.0	96.10	3.31
	1	fl oz							
evaporated, whole	100.0	g	134	6.8	10.0	106.0	303.0	203.0	7.56
	31.5	g	42	2.1	3.2	33.4	95.40	63.90	2.38
	1	fl oz							
malted	100.0	g	64	3.2	8.7	60.0	150.0	98.00	1.91
	256.0	g	164	8.2	22.2	154.0	384.0	251.0	4.89
	1	c							
chocolate	100.0	g	67	3.4	13.5	79.0	182.0	101.0	0.00
	248.0	g	166	8.4	33.4	196.0	451.0	250.0	0.00
	1	c							
strawberry (whole milk)	100.0	g	85	3.0	11.8	38.0	139.0	94.00	2.97
	248.0	g	211	7.5	29.3	94.2	345.0	233.0	7.37
	1	c							

MILK

	SERVING QUANTITY	SERVING UNIT	CALORIES (kCal)	PROTEIN (g)	TOTAL CARBOHYDRATES (g)	SODIUM (mg)	POTASSIUM (mg)	PHOSPHORUS (mg)	TOTAL FAT (g)
SOY	100.0	g	43	2.6	4.9	47.0	122.0	43.00	1.47
	244.0	g	105	6.3	12.0	115.0	298.0	105.0	3.59
	1	c							
soy, light	100.0	g	30	2.4	3.5	48.0	117.0	87.00	0.77
	244.0	g	73	5.8	8.6	117.0	285.0	212.0	1.88
	1	c							
soy, chocolate	100.0	g	63	2.3	10.0	53.0	143.0	51.00	1.53
	244.0	g	154	5.5	24.3	129.0	349.0	124.0	3.73
	1	c							
soy, non-fat	100.0	g	28	2.5	4.1	57.0	105.0	87.00	0.04
	244.0	g	68	6.0	10.1	139.0	256.0	212.0	0.10
	1	c							
RICE	100.0	g	47	0.3	9.2	39.0	27.00	56.00	0.97
	244.0	g	115	0.7	22.4	95.2	65.90	137.0	2.37
	1	c							
rice milk, unsweetened	100.0	g	47	0.3	9.2	39.0	27.00	56.00	0.97
	240.0	g	113	0.7	22.0	93.6	64.80	134.0	2.33
	8	fl oz							
ALMOND, unsweetened	100.0	g	15	0.4	1.3	72.0	67.00	9.00	0.96
	244.0	g	37	1.0	3.2	176.0	163.0	22.00	2.34
	1	c							
almond, unsweetened, chocolate	100.0	g	16	0.5	1.5	72.0	71.00	11.00	1.00
	244.0	g	39	1.1	3.6	176.0	173.0	26.80	2.44
	1	c							
almond milk, sweetened	100.0	g	30	0.4	5.2	69.0	64.00	9.00	0.93
	244.0	g	73	0.9	12.8	168.0	156.0	22.00	2.27
	1	c							
almond, sweetened, chocolate	100.0	g	41	0.4	8.3	67.0	67.00	11.00	0.95
	244.0	g	100	1.1	20.4	163.0	163.0	26.80	2.32
	1	c							
COCONUT	100.0	g	31	0.2	2.9	19.0	19.00	0.00	2.08
	244.0	g	76	0.5	7.1	46.4	46.40	0.00	5.08
	1	c							
GOAT, whole	100.0	g	69	3.6	4.5	50.0	204.0	111.0	4.14
	244.0	g	168	8.7	10.9	122.0	498.0	271.0	10.10
	1	c							

MILK SUBSTITUTE

MILK SUBSTITUTE	SERVING QUANTITY	SERVING UNIT	CALORIES (kCal)	PROTEIN (g)	TOTAL CARBOHYDRATES (g)	SODIUM (mg)	POTASSIUM (mg)	PHOSPHORUS (mg)	TOTAL FAT (g)
Non-dairy milk/creamer	100.0	g	29	1.0	3.8	60.0	80.00	19.00	1.17
	30.5	g	9	0.3	1.1	18.3	24.40	5.80	0.36
	1	fl oz							
imitation, non-soy	100.0	g	46	1.6	5.3	55.0	150.0	100.0	2.00
	244.0	g	112	3.9	12.9	134.0	366.0	244.0	4.88
	1	cup							
Kefir	100.0	g	52	3.6	7.5	38.0	159.0	100.0	0.96
	244.0	g	127	8.8	18.3	92.7	388.0	244	2.34
	1	c							
Sorbet	100.0	g	110	0.8	27.1	13.0	28.00	3.00	0.05
	80.0	g	88	0.6	21.7	10.4	22.40	2.40	0.04
	1	bar							

YOGURT

YOGURT	SERVING QUANTITY	SERVING UNIT	CALORIES (kCal)	PROTEIN (g)	TOTAL CARBOHYDRATES (g)	SODIUM (mg)	POTASSIUM (mg)	PHOSPHORUS (mg)	TOTAL FAT (g)
coconut milk, yogurt	100.0	g	64	0.3	8.0	21.0	27.00	2.00	3.50
	170.0	g	109	0.5	13.5	35.7	45.90	3.40	5.95
	6	oz							
dressing	100.0	g	220	3.5	11.8	43.0	146.0	85.00	18.27
	15.4	g	34	0.5	1.8	6.6	22.50	13.10	2.81
	1	tbsp							
liquid	100.0	g	72	3.7	11.8	53.0	171.0	103.0	1.09
	245.0	g	176	9.1	28.9	130.0	419.0	252.0	2.67
	1	c							
plain, whole milk	100.0	g	61	3.5	4.7	46.0	155.0	95.00	3.25
	227.0	g	138	7.9	10.6	104.0	352.0	216.0	7.38
	8	oz							
	100.0	g	87	3.1	12.4	44.0	146.0	86.00	2.87
Whole milk with fruit	170.0	g	14 8	5.3	21.0	74.8	248.0	146.0	4.88
	6	oz							

YOGURT	SERVING QUANTITY	SERVING UNIT	CALORIES (kCal)	PROTEIN (g)	TOTAL CARBOHYDRATES (g)	SODIUM (mg)	POTASSIUM (mg)	PHOSPHORUS (mg)	TOTAL FAT (g)
whole milk, flavored (non-fruit)	100.0	g	77	3.3	9.4	44.0	147.0	90.00	3.10
	170.0	g	131	5.6	16.0	74.8	250.0	153.0	5.27
	6	oz							
non-fat milk, plain,vanilla	100.0	g	78	2.9	17.0	47.0	141.0	88.00	0.00
	227.0	g	177	6.7	38.7	107.0	320.0	200.0	0.00
	8	oz							
non-fat milk, fruit	100.0	g	83	5.1	15.0	72.0	234.0	140.0	0.17
	170.0	g	141	8.7	25.5	122.0	398.0	238.0	0.29
	6	oz							
Soy, yogurt, plain	100.0	g	94	3.5	16.0	35.0	47.00	38.00	1.80
	170.0	g	160	6.0	27.1	59.5	79.90	64.60	3.06
	6	oz							
Greek, plain, whole milk	100.0	g	97	9.0	4.0	35.0	141.0	135.0	5.00
	170.0	g	165	15.3	6.8	59.5	240.0	230.0	8.50
	6	oz							
Greek, fruit, whole milk	100.0	g	106	7.3	12.3	37.0	113.0	109.0	3.00
	170.0	g	180	12.5	20.9	62.9	192.0	185.0	5.10
	6	oz							
Greek, flavored, other than fruit	100.0	g	111	8.5	9.4	39.0	121.0	117.0	4.44
	170.0	g	189	14.4	15.9	66.3	206.0	199.0	7.55
	6	oz							
Greek, plain, low fat	100.0	g	73	10.0	3.9	34.0	141.0	137.0	1.92
	170.0	g	124	16.9	6.7	57.8	240.0	233.0	3.26
	6	oz							
Greek, LF, flavors other than fruit	100.0	g	95	8.6	9.5	40.0	123.0	119.0	2.50
	170.0	g	162	14.7	16.2	68.0	209.0	202.0	4.25
	6	oz							
Greek, non-fat (NF), plain	100.0	g	59	10.2	3.6	36.0	141.0	135.0	0.39
	170.0	g	100	17.3	6.1	61.2	240.0	230.0	0.66
	6	oz							
Greek, NF, flavors other than fruit	100.0	g	78	8.6	10.4	34.0	123.0	119.0	0.18
	170.0	g	133	14.7	17.6	57.8	209.0	202.0	0.31
	6	oz							
Frozen yogurt, chocolate	100.0	g	131	3.0	21.6	63.0	234.0	89.00	3.60
	160.0	g	210	4.8	34.6	101.0	374.0	142.0	5.76
1 scoop= small cup	1	scoop							

YOGURT

	SERVING QUANTITY	SERVING UNIT	CALORIES (KCal)	PROTEIN (g)	TOTAL CARBOHYDRATES (g)	SODIUM (mg)	POTASSIUM (mg)	PHOSPHORUS (mg)	TOTAL FAT (g)
Frozen yogurt, ***vanilla***	100.0	g	127	3.0	21.6	63.0	156.0	89.00	3.60
	160.0	g	203	4.8	34.6	101.0	250.0	142.0	5.76
1 scoop= small cup	1	scoop							
Frozen yogurt, soft serve, ***chocolate***	100.0	g	160	4.3	24.9	86.0	237.0	141.0	5.76
	175.0	g	280	7.5	43.5	150.0	415.0	247.0	10.10
	1	c							
Frozn yogurt, soft serve, ***vanilla***	100.0	g	159	4.0	24.2	87.0	211.0	129.0	5.60
	175.0	g	278	7.0	42.4	152.0	369.0	226.0	9.80
	1	c							
Frozn yogurt bar, ***vanilla***	100.0	g	127	3.0	21.6	63.0	156.0	89.00	3.60
	65.0	g	83	2.0	14.0	41.0	101.0	57.80	2.34
	1	bar							
Frozn yogurt bar, ***chocolate***	100.0	g	131	3.0	21.6	63.0	234.0	89.00	3.60
	65.0	g	85	2.0	14.0	41.0	152.0	57.80	2.34
	1	bar							
Frozn yogurt cone, ***vanilla***	100.0	g	139	3.2	23.9	71.0	154.0	89.00	3.73
	125.0	g	174	4.0	29.9	88.8	192.0	111.0	4.66
	1	cone							
Frozn yogurt cone, ***chocolate***	100.0	g	142	3.2	23.9	71.0	229.0	89.00	3.73
	125.0	g	178	4.0	29.9	88.8	286.0	111.0	4.66
	1	cone							
Frozn yogurt, ***waffle*** *cone,* ***vanilla***	100.0	g	143	3.3	25.3	77.0	155.0	90.00	3.61
	255.0	g	365	8.4	64.5	196.0	395.0	230.0	9.20
	1	cone							
Frozn yogurt, ***waffle*** *cone,* ***choco***	100.0	g	147	3.3	25.3	77.0	229.0	90.00	3.61
	255.0	g	375	8.4	64.5	196.0	584.0	230.0	9.20
	1	cone							

CHEESE

CHEESE	SERVING QUANTITY	SERVING UNIT	CALORIES (kCal)	PROTEIN (g)	TOTAL CARBOHYDRATES (g)	SODIUM (mg)	POTASSIUM (mg)	PHOSPHORUS (mg)	TOTAL FAT (g)
mozzarella, from whole milk	100.0	g	299	22.2	2.4	486.0	76.00	354.0	22.14
shredded	112.0	g	335	24.8	2.7	544.0	85.10	396.0	24.80
	1	c							
mozzarella, part skim milk	100.0	g	254	24.3	2.8	619.0	84.00	463.0	15.92
	28.35	g	72	6.9	0.8	175.0	23.80	131.0	4.51
	1	oz							
Mozzarella, reduced sodium	100.0	g	280	27.5	3.1	16.0	95.00	524.0	17.10
(shredded)	113.0	g	316	31.1	3.5	18.1	107.0	592.0	19.30
	1	cup							
ricotta, from whole milk	100.0	g	158	7.8	6.9	105.0	230.0	162.0	11.00
	129.0	g	204	10.1	8.9	135.0	297.0	209.0	14.20
	0.5	c							
riccota, part skim milk	100.0	g	138	11.4	5.1	99.0	125.0	183.0	7.91
	124.0	g	171	14.1	6.4	123.0	155.0	227.0	9.81
	0.5	c							
cream cheese, regular	100.0	g	295	7.1	3.5	436.0	112.0	91.00	28.60
	28.35	g	84	2.0	1.0	124.0	31.80	25.80	8.11
	1	oz							
cream cheese, light	100.0	g	201	7.9	8.1	359.0	247.0	152.0	15.28
	28.35	g	57	2.2	2.3	102.0	70.00	43.10	4.33
	1	oz							
processed cheese food	100.0	g	307	16.1	8.9	1279.0	295.0	768.0	23.06
	21.0	g	65	3.4	1.9	269.0	62.00	161.0	4.84
	1	slice							
Cottage cheese	100.0	g	84	11.0	4.3	321.0	120.0	148.0	2.30
	210.0	g	176	23.1	9.1	674.0	252.0	311.0	4.83
	1	cup							
cottage cheese. low fat	100.0	g	84	11.0	4.3	321.0	120.0	148.0	2.30
	226.0	g	190	24.9	9.7	725.0	271.0	334.0	5.20
	1	cup							
Monterey shredded	100.0	g	373	24.5	0.7	600.0	81.00	444.0	30.28
	113.0	g	421	27.7	0.8	678.0	91.50	502.0	34.20
	1	cup							
Cheddar	100.0	g	408	23.3	2.4	654.0	77.00	458.0	34.00
	21.0	g	86	4.9	0.5	137.0	16.20	96.20	7.14
	1	slice							

CHEESE

CHEESE	SERVING QUANTITY	SERVING UNIT	CALORIES (kCal)	PROTEIN (g)	TOTAL CARBOHYDRATES (g)	SODIUM (mg)	POTASSIUM (mg)	PHOSPHORUS (mg)	TOTAL FAT (g)
Cheddar, reduced sodium	100.0	g	398	24.4	1.9	21.0	112.0	484.0	32.62
	21.0	g	84	5.1	0.4	4.4	23.50	102.0	6.85
	1	slice							
Cheddar, sharp sliced	100.0	g	410	24.3	2.1	644.0	76.00	460.0	33.82
	28.0	g	115	6.8	0.6	180.0	21.30	129.0	9.47
	1	oz							
Cheddar/ American cheese spread	100.0	g	290	16.4	8.7	1625	242.0	875.0	21.23
	21.0	g	61	3.5	1.8	341.0	50.80	184.0	4.46
	1	wedge							
American	100.0	g	307	16.1	8.9	1279.	295.0	768.0	23.06
	21.0	g	65	3.4	1.9	269.0	62.00	161.0	4.84
	1	slice							
Brick	100.0	g	371	23.2	2.8	560.0	136.0	451.0	29.68
	17.2	g	64	4.0	0.5	96.3	23.40	77.60	5.10
	1	cubic inch							
Brie	100.0	g	334	20.8	0.5	629.0	152.0	188.0	27.68
	17.0	g	57	3.5	0.1	107.0	25.80	32.00	4.71
	1	cubic inch							
blue	100.0	g	353	21.4	2.3	1146	256.0	387.0	28.74
	28.35	g	100	6.1	0.7	325.0	72.60	110.0	8.15
	1	oz							
Camembert	100.0	g	300	19.8	0.5	842.0	187.0	347.0	24.26
	38.0	g	114	7.5	0.2	320.0	71.10	132.0	9.22
1 wedge = 1.33 oz	1	wedge							
Colby	100.0	g	394	23.8	2.6	604.0	127.0	457.0	32.11
	21.0	g	83	5.0	0.5	127.0	26.70	96.00	6.74
	1	slice							
Caraway	100.0	g	376	25.2	1.1	690.0	93.00	490.0	29.20
	28.35	g	107	7.1	0.9	196.0	26.40	139.0	8.28
	1	oz							
Edam	100.0	g	356	24.9	2.2	819.0	121.0	546.0	27.44
	21.0	g	75	5.2	0.5	172.0	25.40	115.0	5.76
	1	slice							
Feta	100.0	g	265	14.2	3.9	1139.	62.00	337.0	21.49
	17.0	g	45	2.4	0.7	194.0	10.50	57.30	3.62
	1	cubic inch							
Fontina	100.0	g	389	25.6	1.6	800.0	64.00	346.0	31.14
	21.0	g	82	5.4	0.3	168.0	13.40	72.70	6.54
	1	Slice							
goat	100.0	g	364	21.6	0.1	415.0	158.0	375.0	29.84
	25.0	g	91	5.4	0.0	104.0	39.50	93.80	7.46
	1	cubic inch							

CHEESE	SERVING QUANTITY	SERVING UNIT	CALORIES (KCal)	PROTEIN (g)	TOTAL CARBOHYDRATES (g)	SODIUM (mg)	POTASSIUM (mg)	PHOSPHORUS (mg)	TOTAL FAT (g)
Gouda	100.0	g	356	24.9	2.2	819.0	121.0	546.0	27.44
	28.35	g	101	7.0	0.6	232.0	34.30	155.0	7.78
	1	oz							
Gruyere	100.0	g	413	29.8	0.4	714.0	81.00	605.0	32.34
	21.0	g	87	6.3	0.1	150.0	17.00	127.0	6.70
	1	slice							
Blue or	100.0	g	353	21.4	2.3	1146.0	256.0	387.0	28.74
Roquefort	17.3	g	61	3.7	0.4	198.0	44.30	67.00	4.97
	1	cubic inch							
Colby Jack	100.0	g	384	24.1	1.6	602.0	104.0	450.0	31.20
	21.0	g	81	5.1	0.3	126.0	21.80	94.50	6.55
	1	slice							
Parmesan,	100.0	g	420	29.6	12.4	1750.0	184.0	634.0	28.00
grated	7.6	g	32	2.3	0.9	133.0	14.00	48.20	1.82
	1	tbsp							
Parmesan,	100.0	g	421	29.6	12.4	1750.0	184.0	634.0	28.00
hard	10.3	g	43	3.1	1.3	180.0	19.00	65.30	2.88
	1	cubic inch							
Mexican blend	100.0	g	358	23.5	1.8	607.0	85.00	438.0	28.51
shredded	113.0	g	405	26.6	2.0	686.0	96.00	495.0	32.20
	1	cup							
Mexican blend,	100.0	g	282	24.7	3.4	776.0	93.00	583.0	19.40
reduced fat shredded	113.0	g	319	27.9	3.9	877.0	105.0	659.0	21.90
	1	cup							
Muenster	100.0	g	368	23.4	1.1	628.0	134.0	468.0	30.04
	21.0	g	77	5.0	0.2	132.0	28.10	98.30	6.31
	1	slice							
Neufchatel	100.0	g	253	9.2	3.6	334.0	152.0	138.0	22.78
	28.35	g	72	2.6	1.0	94.7	43.10	39.10	6.46
	1	oz							
Provolone	100.0	g	351	25.6	2.1	727.0	138.0	496.0	26.62
	21.0	g	74	5.4	0.4	153.0	29.00	104.0	5.59
	1	slice							
Romano	100.0	g	387	31.8	3.6	1433.0	86.00	760.0	26.94
	28.35	g	110	9.0	1.0	406.0	24.40	215.0	7.64
	1	oz							
Swiss	100.0	g	393	27.0	1.4	185.0	71.00	574.0	31.00
	21.0	g	83	5.7	0.3	38.8	14.90	121.0	6.51
	1	slice							
Tilsiter/ Tilsit	100.0	g	340	24.4	1.9	753.0	65.00	500.0	25.98
	28.35	g	96	6.9	0.5	213.0	18.40	142.0	7.36
	1	oz							

CREAM

CREAM	SERVING QUANTITY	SERVING UNIT	CALORIES (kCal)	PROTEIN (g)	TOTAL CARBOHYDRATES (g)	SODIUM (mg)	POTASSIUM (mg)	PHOSPHORUS (mg)	TOTAL FAT (g)
sour cream, regular	100.0	g	198	2.4	4.6	31.0	125.0	76.00	19.35
	30.0	g	59	0.7	1.4	9.3	37.50	22.80	5.80
	1	container							
sour cream, light	100.0	g	136	3.5	7.1	83.0	212.0	71.00	10.60
	240.0	g	326	8.4	17.0	199.0	509.0	170.0	25.40
	1	cup							
sour cream, imitation	100.0	g	208	2.4	6.6	102.0	161.0	45.00	19.52
	240.0	g	499	5.8	15.9	245.0	386.0	108.0	46.80
	1	cup							
sour cream, fat free	100.0	g	74	3.1	15.6	141.0	129.0	95.00	0.00
	240.0	g	178	7.4	37.4	338.0	310.0	228.0	0.00
	1	cup							
heavy full cream	100.0	g	340	2.8	2.8	27.0	95.00	58.00	36.08
	30.0	g	102	0.9	1.0	8.1	28.50	17.40	10.80
	1	fl oz							
whipped	100.0	g	343	2.7	8.6	26.0	89.00	55.00	33.94
	40.0	g	137	1.1	3.4	10.4	35.60	22.00	13.60
	1	cup							
half and half	100.0	g	131	3.1	4.3	61.0	132.0	95.00	11.50
	30.0	g	39	0.9	1.3	18.3	39.60	28.50	3.45
	1	fl oz							
coffee, light cream	100.0	g	195	3.0	3.7	72.0	136.0	92.00	19.10
	11.0	g	21	0.3	0.4	7.9	15.00	10.10	2.10
	1	ind. container							

F. Fats

(Oils, Nuts, & Seeds)

Hey there!

Do you need to print out this Food List?

You can download a printable version of this chart by scanning the QR code below or copying the link on your computer browser.

ALMOND	SERVING QUANTITY	SERVING UNIT	CALORIES (kCal)	PROTEIN (g)	TOTAL CARBOHYDRATES (g)	SODIUM (mg)	POTASSIUM (mg)	PHOSPHORUS (mg)	TOTAL FAT (g)
whole	100.0	g	579	21.2	21.6	1.00	733.0	481.0	49.9
	35.75	g	207	7.6	7.7	0.36	262.0	171.9	17.9
	0.25	c							
slivered	100.0	g	579	21.2	21.6	1.00	733.0	481.0	49.9
	27.0	g	156	5.7	5.8	0.27	197.9	129.8	13.5
	0.25	c							
ground	100.0	g	579	21.2	21.6	1.00	733.0	481.0	49.9
	23.75	g	138	5.0	5.1	0.24	174.1	114.4	11.9
	0.25	c							
paste (marzipan)	100.0	g	458	9.0	47.8	9.00	314.0	258.0	27.7
	28.38	g	130	2.6	13.6	2.55	89.10	73.21	7.9
	2	tbsp							
oil	100.0	g	884	0.0	0.0	0.00	0.00	0.00	100.0
	13.6	g	120	0.0	0.0	0.00	0.00	0.00	13.6
	1	tbsp							
butter, without salt added	100.0	g	614	21.0	18.8	227.0	748.0	508.0	55.5
	16.0	g	98	3.4	3.0	1.12	119.6	81.28	8.9
	1	tbsp							
dry roasted, without salt added	100.0	g	598	3.0	21.0	3.00	713.0	471.0	52.5
	34.5	g	206	7.2	7.3	1.04	246.0	162.5	18.1
	0.25	c							
oil roasted, without salt	100.0	g	607	21.2	17.7	1.00	699.0	466.0	55.2
	39.25	g	238	8.3	6.9	0.39	274.3	182.9	21.7
	0.25	c							
milk, unsweetened, *shelf stable*	100.0	g	15	0.4	1.3	72.00	67.00	9.00	1.0
	262.0	g	39	1.1	3.4	188.6	175.5	23.58	2.5
	1	c							
milk, sweetened, *vanilla flavor ready-to-drink*	100.0	g	38	0.4	6.6	63.00	50.00	8.00	1.0
	240.0	g	91	1.0	15.8	151.2	120.0	19.20	2.5
	1	c							
milk, chocolate *flavor, unsweetened fortified Vit. D2 and E*	100.0	g	21	0.8	1.3	75.00	96.00	17.00	1.5
	240.0	g	50	2.0	3.0	180.0	130.4	40.80	3.5
	1	c							

WALNUT	SERVING QUANTITY	SERVING UNIT	CALORIES (kCal)	PROTEIN (g)	TOTAL CARBOHYDRATES (g)	SODIUM (mg)	POTASSIUM (mg)	PHOSPHORUS (mg)	TOTAL FAT (g)
english, halves	100.0	g	654	15.2	13.7	2.00	441.0	346.0	65.2
	25.0	g	164	3.8	3.4	0.50	110.2	86.50	16.3
	0.25	c							
english, ground	100.0	g	654	15.2	13.7	2.00	441.0	346.0	65.2
	20.0	g	131	3.1	2.7	0.40	88.20	69.20	13.0
	0.25	c							
english, chopped	100.0	g	654	15.2	13.7	2.00	441.0	346.0	65.2
	29.25	g	191	4.5	4.0	0.59	129.0	101.2	19.1
	0.25	c							
butternut or white walnut, dried	100.0	g	612	24.9	12.1	1.00	421.0	446.0	57.0
	120.0	g	734	29.9	14.5	1.20	505.2	535.2	68.4
	1	c							
black or american, dried, chopped	100.0	g	619	24.1	9.6	2.00	523.0	513.0	59.3
	31.25	g	193	7.5	3.0	0.63	163.4	160.3	18.5
	0.25	c							
black or american, dried, ground	100.0	g	604	23.5	9.3	1.95	509.9	500.2	57.9
	26.67	g	161	6.3	2.5	0.52	135.9	133.4	15.4
	0.33	c							
glazed	100.0	g	500	8.3	47.6	446.0	232.0	na	35.7
	28.35	g	142	2.4	13.5	126.5	65.77	na	10.1
	1	oz							
oil	100.0	g	884	0.0	0.0	0.0	0.00	0.00	100.0
	13.6	g	120	0.0	0.0	0.0	0.00	0.00	13.6
	1	tbsp							

PECANS	SERVING QUANTITY	SERVING UNIT	CALORIES (kCal)	PROTEIN (g)	TOTAL CARBOHYDRATES (g)	SODIUM (mg)	POTASSIUM (mg)	PHOSPHORUS (mg)	TOTAL FAT (g)
chopped	100.0	g	691	9.2	13.9	0.00	410.0	277.0	72.0
	109.0	g	753	10.0	15.1	0.00	446.9	410.0	78.5
	1	c							
halves	100.0	g	691	9.2	13.9	0.00	410.0	277.0	72.0
	24.75	g	171	2.3	3.4	0.00	101.4	68.56	17.8
	0.25	c							
halves, oil roasted	100.0	g	715	9.2	13.0	1.00	392.0	263.0	75.2
	110.0	g	787	10.1	14.3	1.10	431.2	289.3	82.8
	1	c							
dry roasted, without salt added	100.0	g	710	9.5	13.6	1.00	424.0	293.0	74.3
	28.35	g	201	2.7	3.8	0.28	120.2	83.07	21.1
	1	oz							
PISTACHIO									
raw	100.0	g	560	20.2	27.2	1.00	1,025	490.0	45.3
(1 oz = 49 kernels)	123.0	g	689	24.8	33.4	1.23	1,261	602.7	55.7
	1	c							
dry roasted, no salt added	100.0	g	572	21.1	28.3	6.00	1,007	469.0	45.8
	123.0	g	704	25.9	34.8	7.38	1,239	576.8	56.4
	1	c							
MACADAMIA									
whole or halves	100.0	g	718	7.9	13.8	5.00	368.0	188.0	75.8
(1 oz = 10-12 kernels)	134.0	g	962	10.6	18.5	6.70	493.1	251.9	101.5
	1	c							
dry roasted, without salt added	100.0	g	718	7.8	13.4	4.00	363.0	198.0	76.1
	33.5.0	g	241	2.6	4.5	1.34	121.6	66.33	25.5
	0.25	c							

CASHEW	SERVING QUANTITY	SERVING UNIT	CALORIES (kCal)	PROTEIN (g)	TOTAL CARBOHYDRATES (g)	SODIUM (mg)	POTASSIUM (mg)	PHOSPHORUS (mg)	TOTAL FAT (g)
raw	100.0	g	553	18.2	30.2	12.00	660.0	593.0	43.9
	28.35	g	157	5.2	8.6	3.40	187.1	168.1	12.4
	1	oz							
oil roasted, no salt added	100.0	g	580	16.8	29.9	13.00	632.0	531.0	47.8
	129.0	g	748	21.7	38.5	16.77	815.2	685	61.6
	1	c							
dry roasted, no salt aded	100.0	g	574	15.3	32.7	16.00	565.0	490.0	46.4
(halves and whole)	137.0	g	786	21.0	44.8	21.92	774.0	671.3	63.5
	1	c							
butter, without salt added	100.0	g	587	17.6	27.6	15.00	546.0	457.0	49.4
	32.0	g	188	5.6	8.8	4.80	174.7	146.3	15.8
	2	tbsp							
HAZELNUT									
oil	100.0	g	884	0.0	0.0	0.00	0.00	0.00	100.0
	13.6	g	120	0.0	0.0	0.00	0.00	0.00	13.6
	1	tbsp							
whole (1 oz= 21 kernels)	100.0	g	628	15.0	16.7	0.00	680.0	290.0	60.8
	33.75	g	212	5.1	5.6	0.00	229.5	97.88	20.5
	0.25	c							
blanched	100.0	g	629	13.7	17.0	0.00	658.0	310.0	61.2
	28.35	g	178	3.9	4.8	0.00	186.5	87.89	17.3
	1	oz							
chopped	100.0	g	628	15.0	16.7	0.00	680.0	290.0	60.8
	28.75	g	181	4.3	4.8	0.00	195.5	83.38	17.5
	0.25	c							
ground	100.0	g	628	15.0	16.7	0.00	680.0	290.0	60.8
	18.75	g	118	2.8	3.1	0.00	127.5	54.38	11.4
	0.25	c							
dry roasted, without salt added	100.0	g	646	15.0	17.6	0.00	755.0	310.0	62.4
	28.35	g	183	4.3	5.0	0.00	214.0	87.89	17.7
	1	oz							
spread, chocolate flavored	100.0	g	539	5.4	62.4	41.00	407.0	152.0	29.7

PEANUT	SERVING QUANTITY	SERVING UNIT	CALORIES (kCal)	PROTEIN (g)	TOTAL CARBOHYDRATES (g)	SODIUM (mg)	POTASSIUM (mg)	PHOSPHORUS (mg)	TOTAL FAT (g)
oil	100.0	g	884	0.0	0.0	0.00	0.00	0.00	100.0
	13.5	g	119	0.0	0.0	0.00	0.00	0.00	13.5
	1	tbsp							
all types	100.0	g	567	25.8	16.1	18.00	705.0	376.0	49.2
	36.5	g	207	9.4	5.9	6.57	257.3	137.2	18.0
	0.25	c							
all types, dry roasted, no salt added	100.0	g	587	24.4	21.4	6.00	634.0	363.0	49.7
(1 Oz = 28.35g)	36.5	g	214	8.9	7.8	2.19	231.4	132.5	18.1
	0.25	c							
all types, oil roasted, no salt	100.0	g	599	28.0	15.3	6.00	726.0	397.0	52.5
	133.0	g	797	37.3	20.3	7.98	965.5	528.0	69.8
	1	c							
butter, smooth, reduced fat	100.0	g	520	25.9	36.7	540.0	669.0	369.0	34.0
	36.0	g	187	9.3	12.8	194.4	240.8	132.8	12.2
	2	tbsp							
butter, smooth, no salt added	100.0	g	598	22.2	22.3	17.00	558.0	335.0	51.4
	32.0	g	191	7.1	7.1	5.44	178.5	107.2	16.4
	2	tbsp							
butter, chunky, no salt added	100.0	g	589	24.1	21.6	17.00	745.0	319.0	49.9
	32.0	g	188	7.7	6.9	5.44	238.4	102.0	16.0
	2	tbsp							
butter, reduced sodium	100.0	g	590	24.0	21.8	203.0	747.0	317.0	49.9
	16.0	g	94	3.8	3.5	32.48	119.5	50.72	8.0
	1	tbsp							
sauce, made with PB, water & soy sauce	100.0	g	257	6.3	22.0	1338	235.0	107.0	16.0
	18.0	g	46	1.1	4.0	240.8	42.30	19.26	2.9
	1	tbsp							
brittle	100.0	g	486	7.6	71.2	445.0	168.0	106.0	19.0
	42.53	g	207	3.2	30.3	189.2	71.44	45.08	8.1
	1.5	oz							
flour, defatted	100.0	g	327	52.2	34.7	180.0	1,290	760.0	0.6
	30.0	g	98	15.7	10.4	54.00	387.0	228.0	0.2
	0.5	c							

PINE	SERVING QUANTITY	SERVING UNIT	CALORIES (kCal)	PROTEIN (g)	TOTAL CARBOHYDRATES (g)	SODIUM (mg)	POTASSIUM (mg)	PHOSPHORUS (mg)	TOTAL FAT (g)
(Pinyon), dried	100.0	g	629	11.6	19.3	72.00	628.0	35.00	61.0
	28.35	g	178	3.3	5.5	20.41	178.0	9.92	17.3
	1	oz							
(Pignolia), dried	100.0	g	673	13.7	13.1	2.00	597.0	575.0	68.4
	8.6	g	58	1.2	1.1	0.17	51.34	49.45	5.9
	1	tbsp							
CHESTNUT									
Japanese	100.0	g	154	2.3	34.9	14.00	329.0	72.00	0.5
	28.35	g	44	0.6	9.9	3.97	93.27	20.41	0.2
	1	oz							
Chinese	100.0	g	224	4.2	49.1	3.00	447.0	96.00	1.1
	28.35	g	64	1.2	13.9	0.85	126.7	27.22	0.3
	1	oz							
European, unpeeled	100.0	g	213	2.4	45.5	3.00	518.0	93.00	2.3
	36.25	g	77	0.9	16.5	1.09	187.7	33.71	0.8
	0.25	c							
European, peeled	100.0	g	196	1.6	44.2	2.00	484.0	38.00	1.3
	28.35	g	56	0.5	12.5	0.57	137.2	10.77	0.4
	1	oz							
European, roasted	100.0	g	245	3.2	53.0	2.00	592.0	107.0	2.2
	28.35	g	69	0.9	15.0	0.57	167.8	30.33	0.6
	1	oz							
Japanese, roasted	100.0	g	201	3.0	45.1	19.00	427.0	93.00	0.8
	28.35	g	57	0.8	12.8	5.39	121.0	26.37	0.2
	1	oz							
Chinese, roasted	100.0	g	239	4.5	52.4	4.00	477.0	102.0	1.2
	28.35	g	68	1.3	14.8	1.13	135.2	28.92	0.3
	1	oz							
Chinese, boiled and steamed	100.0	g	153	2.9	33.6	2.00	306.0	66.00	0.8
	28.35	g	43	0.8	9.5	0.57	86.75	18.71	0.2
	1	oz							
European, boiled and steamed	100.0	g	131	2.0	27.8	27.00	715.0	99.00	1.4
	28.35	g	37	0.6	7.9	7.65	202.7	15.31	0.4
	1	oz							
Japanese, boiled and steamed	100.0	g	56	0.8	12.6	5.00	119.0	26.00	0.2
	28.35	g	16	0.2	3.6	1.42	33.74	7.37	0.1
	1	oz							

ACORN	SERVING QUANTITY	SERVING UNIT	CALORIES (kCal)	PROTEIN (g)	TOTAL CARBOHYDRATES (g)	SODIUM (mg)	POTASSIUM (mg)	PHOSPHORUS (mg)	TOTAL FAT (g)
Nuts	100.0	g	387	6.2	40.8	0.00	539.0	79.00	23.9
	28.35	g	110	1.7	11.6	0.00	152.8	22.40	6.8
	1	oz							
flour	100.0	g	501	7.5	54.7	0.00	712.0	103.0	30.2
	28.35	g	142	2.1	15.5	0.00	201.8	29.20	8.6
	1	oz							
nuts, dried	100.0	g	509	8.1	53.7	0.00	709.0	103.0	31.4
	28.35	g	144	2.3	15.2	0.00	201.0	29.20	8.9
	1	oz							
CHIA									
seeds, dried	100.0	g	486	16.5	42.1	16.00	407.0	860.0	30.7
	28.35	g	138	4.7	11.9	4.54	115.3	243.8	8.7
	1	oz							
HEMP									
seeds, hulled	100.0	g	553	31.6	8.7	5.00	1,200	1,650	48.8
	30.0	g	166	9.5	2.6	1.50	360.0	495.0	14.6
	3	tbsp							
FLAXSEED									
seeds, whole	100.0	g	534	18.3	28.9	30.00	813.0	642.0	42.2
	10.3	g	55	1.9	3.0	3.09	83.70	66.10	4.3
	1	tbsp							
seeds, ground	7.0	g	37	1.3	2.0	2.10	56.90	44.90	3.0
	1	tbsp							
oil	100.0	g	884	0.1	0.0	0.00	0.00	1.00	100.0
	14.0	g	124	0.0	0.0	0.00	0.00	0.14	14.0
	1	tbsp							
oil with added sliced flaxseed	100.0	g	878	0.4	0.4	6.00	31.00	27.00	99.0
	13.7	g	120	0.1	0.1	0.82	4.25	3.70	13.6
	1	tbsp							
oil, cold pressed	100.0	g	884	0.1	0.0	0.00	0.00	1.00	100.0
	13.6	g	120	0.0	0.0	0.00	0.00	0.14	13.6
	1	tbsp							

SESAME	SERVING QUANTITY	SERVING UNIT	CALORIES (kCal)	PROTEIN (g)	TOTAL CARBOHYDRATES (g)	SODIUM (mg)	POTASSIUM (mg)	PHOSPHORUS (mg)	TOTAL FAT (g)
seeds, kernels, toasted	100	g	567	17.0	26.0	39.00	406.0	774.0	48.0
	128	g	726	21.7	33.3	49.92	519.6	990.7	61.4
	1	c							
butter or Tahini	100	g	592	17.4	21.5	35.00	459.0	790.0	53.0
	30	g	178	5.2	6.5	10.50	137.7	237.0	15.9
	2	tbsp							
seeds, whole, dried	100	g	573	17.7	23.5	11.00	468.0	629.0	49.7
	9	g	52	1.6	2.1	0.99	42.12	56.61	4.5
	1	tbsp							
butter or Tahini, from roasted/toasted kernels	100	g	595	17.0	21.2	115.0	414.0	732.0	53.8
	30	g	179	5.1	6.4	34.50	124.2	219.6	16.1
	2	tbsp							
SUNFLOWER									
seeds, kernels, toasted	100	g	619	17.2	20.6	3.00	491.0	1,158	56.8
	33.5	g	207	5.8	6.9	1.01	164.5	387.9	19.0
	0.25	c							
seeds, kernels, dried	100	g	584	20.8	20.0	9.00	645.0	660.0	51.5
	36	g	210	7.5	7.2	3.24	232.2	237.6	18.5
	0.25	c							
seeds, kernels, oil roasted	100	g	592	20.1	22.9	3.00	483.0	1,139	51.3
	135	g	799	27.1	31.0	4.05	652.0	1,538	69.3
	1	c							
seeds, kernel. dry roasted	100	g	582	19.3	24.1	3.00	850.0	1,155	49.8
	32	g	186	6.2	7.7	0.96	272.0	369.6	15.9
	0.25	c							
butter, without salt added	100	g	617	17.3	23.3	3.00	576.0	666.0	55.2
	16	g	99	2.8	3.7	0.48	92.16	106.5	8.8
	1	tbsp							
oil, <60% / >60%/ >70% Linoleic	100	g	884	0.0	0.0	0.00	0.00	0.00	100.0
	13.6	g	120	0.0	0.0	0.00	0.00	0.00	13.6
	1	tbsp							
oil, industrial, mid-oleic for frying and salad dressings	100	g	884	0.0	0.0	0.00	0.00	0.00	100.0
	13.6	g	120	0.0	0.0	0.00	0.00	0.00	13.6
	1	tbsp							

PUMPKIN	SERVING QUANTITY	SERVING UNIT	CALORIES (KCal)	PROTEIN (g)	TOTAL CARBOHYDRATES (g)	SODIUM (mg)	POTASSIUM (mg)	PHOSPHORUS (mg)	TOTAL FAT (g)
meat, 1" cubes	100.0	g	26	1.0	6.5	1.00	340.0	44.00	0.1
	116.0	g	30	1.2	7.5	1.16	394.4	51.04	0.1
	1	c							
flowers	100.0	g	15	1.0	3.3	5.00	173.0	49.00	0.1
	33.0	g	1	0.0	0.1	0.20	6.92	1.96	0.0
	1	c							
meat, boiled, drained, no salt added	100.0	g	20	0.7	4.9	1.00	230.0	30.00	0.1
	122.5	g	25	0.9	6.0	1.23	281.7	36.75	0.1
	0.5	c							
pumpkin pie spice powder	100.0	g	342	5.8	69.3	52.00	663.0	118.0	12.6
	1.7	g	6	0.1	1.2	0.88	11.27	2.01	0.2
	1	tsp							
seed sunfish, cooked dry heat	100.0	g	114	24.9	0.0	103.0	449.0	231.0	0.9
	85.05	g	97	21.2	0.0	87.60	381.8	196.4	0.8
	3	oz							
seeds, kernels, whole, roasted	100.0	g	446	18.6	53.8	18.00	919.0	92.00	19.4
without salt added	32.0	g	143	5.9	17.2	5.76	294.0	29.44	6.2
	0.5	c							
POPPYSEED									
oil	100.0	g	884	0.0	0.0	0.00	0.00	0.00	100.0
	13.6	g	120	0.0	0.0	0.00	0.00	0.00	13.6
	1	tbsp							
salad dressing, creamy	100.0	g	399	0.9	23.7	933.0	61.00	49.00	33.3
	33.0	g	132	0.3	7.8	307.9	20.13	16.17	11.0
	2	tbsp							

OLIVE

	Serving Quantity	Serving Unit	Calories (kCal)	Protein (g)	Total Carbohydrates (g)	Sodium (mg)	Potassium (mg)	Phosphorus (mg)	Total Fat (g)
oil, extra virgin, virgin	100.0	g	884	0.0	0.0	2.00	1.00	0.00	100.0
	14.0	g	124	0.0	0.0	0.28	0.14	0.00	14.0
	1	Tbsp							
black, kalamata	100.0	g	116	0.8	6.0	735.0	8.00	3.00	10.9
	15.0	g	17	0.1	0.9	110.0	1.20	0.45	1.6
	3	pcs							
green	100.0	g	145	1.0	3.8	1556	42.00	4.00	15.3
	15.0	g	22	0.2	0.6	233.0	6.30	0.60	2.3
	3	pcs							
spread (tapenade)	100.0	g	278	0.7	4.2	835.0	17.00	3.00	30.1
	16.0	g	45	0.1	0.7	134.0	2.72	0.48	4.8
	1	tbsp							
stuffed	100.0	g	128	1.0	4.0	1340	58.00	6.00	13.2
	15.0	g	19	0.2	0.6	201.0	8.70	0.90	2.0
	3	pcs							

COCONUT

	Serving Quantity	Serving Unit	Calories (kCal)	Protein (g)	Total Carbohydrates (g)	Sodium (mg)	Potassium (mg)	Phosphorus (mg)	Total Fat (g)
fresh	100.0	g	354	3.3	15.2	20.00	356.0	113.0	33.5
	85.0	g	301	2.8	12.9	17.00	303.0	96.00	28.5
	1	c							
water, unsweetened	100.0	g	18	0.2	4.2	26.00	165.0	5.00	0.0
	240.0	g	43	0.5	10.2	62.40	396.0	12.00	0.0
	1	c							
milk	100.0	g	31	0.2	2.9	19.00	19.00	0.00	2.1
	244.0	g	76	0.5	7.1	46.40	46.40	0.00	5.1
	1	c							
milk/cream for cooking	100.0	g	230	2.3	5.5	15.00	263.0	100.0	23.8
	240.0	g	552	5.5	13.3	36.00	631.0	240.0	57.2
	1	c							
yogurt	100.0	g	64	0.3	8.0	21.00	27.00	2.00	3.5
	170.0	g	109	0.5	13.5	35.70	45.90	3.40	6.0
	6	oz							
cream, canned, sweetened	100.0	g	357	1.2	53.2	36.00	101.0	22.00	16.3
	37.0	g	132	0.4	19.7	13.30	37.40	8.14	6.0
	¼	c							
oil	100.0	g	833	0.0	0.0	0.00	0.00	0.00	99.1
	14.0	g	117	0.0	0.0	0.00	0.00	0.00	13.9
	1	tbsp							
flaked, shredded, packed	100.0	g	456	3.1	51.9	285.0	361.0	100.0	28.0
	28.0	g	128	1.0	14.5	79.80	101.0	28.00	7.8
	2	tbsp							

	SERVING QUANTITY	SERVING UNIT	CALORIES (kCal)	PROTEIN (g)	TOTAL CARBOHYDRATES (g)	SODIUM (mg)	POTASSIUM (mg)	PHOSPHORUS (mg)	TOTAL FAT (g)
SAFFLOWER									
oil	100.0	g	884	0.0	0.0	0.00	0.00	0.00	100.0
	14.0	g	124	0.0	0.0	0.00	0.00	0.00	14.0
	1	tbsp							
CANOLA									
oil	100.0	g	884	0.0	0.0	0.00	0.00	0.00	100.0
	14.0	g	124	0.0	0.0	0.00	0.00	0.00	14.0
	1	tbsp							
SOYBEAN									
oil	100.0	g	884	0.0	0.0	0.00	0.00	0.00	100.0
	14.0	g	124	0.0	0.0	0.00	0.00	0.00	14.0
	1	tbsp							
BUTTER									
stick	100.0	g	717	0.9	0.1	643.00	24.00	24.00	81.1
	14.0	g	100	0.1	0.0	90.00	3.36	3.36	11.4
	1	tbsp							
light, stick or tub	100.0	g	499	3.3	0.0	450.00	71.00	34.00	55.1
	14.0	g	70	0.5	0.0	63.00	9.94	4.76	7.7
	1	tbsp							
unsalted	100.0	g	717	0.9	0.1	11.00	24.00	24.00	81.1
	14.0	g	102	0.1	0.0	1.56	3.41	3.41	11.5
	1	tbsp							
GHEE									
clarified butter	100.0	g	876	0.3	0.0	2.00	5.00	3.00	99.5
	14.0	g	123	0.0	0.0	0.28	0.70	0.42	13.9
	1	tbsp							
MARGARINE									
stick	100.0	g	717	0.2	0.7	751.00	18.00	5.00	80.7
	14.0	g	100	0.0	0.1	105.00	2.52	0.70	11.3
	1	tbsp							

G. Animal Protein

(Meats, Poultry, and Seafood)

Hey there!

Do you need to print out this Food List?

You can download a printable version of this chart by scanning the QR code below or copying the link on your computer browser.

https://go.renaltracker.com/printfoodlist

SALMON	SERVING QUANTITY	SERVING UNIT	CALORIES (kCal)	PROTEIN (g)	TOTAL CARBOHYDRATES (g)	SODIUM (mg)	POTASSIUM (mg)	PHOSPHORUS (mg)	TOTAL FAT (g)
pink, raw	100.0	g	127	20.5	0.0	74.99	365.9	260.9	4.40
	113.4	g	144	23.2	0.0	85.04	415.0	295.9	4.99
	4.00	oz							
atlantic, wild, raw	100.0	g	142	19.8	0.0	44.00	489.9	199.9	0.98
	113.4	g	161	22.5	0.0	49.89	555.6	226.7	1.11
	4.00	oz							
atlantic, farmed,raw	100.0	g	208	20.4	0.0	58.99	362.9	239.9	13.4
	113.4	g	236	23.2	0.0	66.90	411.6	272.1	15.2
	4.00	oz							
pink, canned, drained solids, w/ bone	100.0	g	138	23.1	0.0	380.78	332.8	378.7	5.02
	85.05	g	117	19.6	0.0	323.85	283.0	322.1	4.27
	3.00	oz							
pink, canned, with bone and liquid no salt	100.0	g	139	19.8	0.0	75.00	326.0	329.0	6.05
	56.70	g	79	11.2	0.0	42.52	184.8	186.5	3.43
	2.00	oz							
pink, canned, drained solids without skin and bones	100.0	g	136	24.6	0.0	378.00	326.0	253.0	4.21
	85.05	g	116	20.9	0.0	321.49	277.2	215.1	3.58
	3.00	oz							
chum, canned, drained, with bone no salt	100.0	g	141	21.4	0.0	75.00	300.0	354.0	5.50
	56.70	g	80	12.2	0.0	42.52	170.1	200.7	3.12
	2.00	oz							
nuggets, breaded, frozen, heated	100.0	g	212	12.7	14	173.00	165.0	176.0	11.7
TUNA									
bluefin, raw	100.0	g	144	23.3	0.0	39.00	251.9	253.9	4.90
	113.4	g	163	26.5	0.0	44.22	285.7	288.0	5.56
	4.00	oz							
yellowfin or Ahi, raw	100.0	g	109	24.4	0.0	45.00	440.9	277.9	0.49
	113.4	g	124	27.7	0.0	51.03	500.0	315.2	0.56
	4.00	oz							
canned in oil, drained, light no salt	100.0	g	198	29.1	0.0	50.00	207.0	311.0	8.21
	56.70	g	112	16.5	0.0	28.35	117.3	176.3	4.65
	2.00	oz							
white, canned in water, drained no salt	100.0	g	128	23.6	0.0	50.00	237.0	217.0	2.97
	56.70	g	73	13.4	0.0	28.35	134.3	123.0	1.68
	2.00	oz							
canned in water, drained, light no salt	100.0	g	116	25.5	0.0	50.00	237.0	163.0	0.82
	56.70	g	66	14.5	0.0	28.35	134.3	92.42	0.46
	2.00	oz							
white, canned in oil, drained, no salt	100.0	g	186	26.5	0.0	50.00	333.0	267.0	8.08
	56.70	g	105	15.0	0.0	28.35	188.8	151.4	4.58
	2.00	oz							

SARDINES	SERVING QUANTITY	SERVING UNIT	CALORIES (kCal)	PROTEIN (g)	TOTAL CARBOHYDRATES (g)	SODIUM (mg)	POTASSIUM (mg)	PHOSPHORUS (mg)	TOTAL FAT (g)
Spanish	100.0	g	212	6.2	14.2	310.0	0.00	na	14.16
	113.0	g	240	7.0	16.0	350.0	0.00	na	16.00
	4.00	oz							
atlantic, canned in oil, with bones	100.0	g	208	24.6	0.0	307.0	397.0	490.0	11.45
	24.00	g	50	5.9	0.0	73.68	95.28	117.6	2.75
	2.00	oz							
portuguese	100.0	g	236	25.5	0.0	500.0	na	na	12.73
	55.00	g	130	14.0	0.0	275.0	na	na	7.00
	0.50	c							
fillets, canned	100.0	g	338	18.2	7.3	364.0	na	na	26.36
	55.00	g	186	10.0	4.0	200.0	na	na	14.50
	0.25	c							
TILAPIA									
raw	100.0	g	96	20.1	0.0	52.00	302.0	170.0	1.70
	113.4	g	107	22.8	0.0	58.97	342.5	192.8	1.93
	4.00	oz							
cooked, dry heat	100.0	g	128	26.2	0.0	55.97	379.8	203.9	2.65
	85.05	g	109	22.2	0.0	47.60	323.0	173.4	2.25
	3.00	oz							
POLLOCK									
atlantic, raw	100.0	g	92	19.4	0.0	85.99	355.9	220.9	0.98
	113.4	g	104	22.0	0.0	97.51	403.7	250.6	1.11
	4.00	oz							
atlantic, cooked, dry heat	100.0	g	118	24.9	0.0	110.0	456.0	283.0	1.26
	85.05	g	100	21.2	0.0	93.55	387.8	240.7	1.07
	3.00	oz							
alaska, untreated, cooked	100.0	g	87	19.4	0.0	166.0	364.0	206.0	1.00
	85.05	g	74	16.5	0.0	141.1	309.6	175.2	0.85
	3.00	oz							
PANGASIUS (CREAM DORY/SWAI)									
fillets, boneless	100.0	g	71	14.2	0.0	186.0	na	na	1.77
	113.0	g	80	16.0	0.0	210.0	na	na	2.00
	4.00	oz							
fillets, skinless, boneless	100.0	g	177	20.4	0.0	52.00	na	na	1.77
	113.0	g	200	23.0	0.0	58.80	na	na	2.00
	4.00	oz							

COD	SERVING QUANTITY	SERVING UNIT	CALORIES (KCal)	PROTEIN (g)	TOTAL CARBOHYDRATES (g)	SODIUM (mg)	POTASSIUM (mg)	PHOSPHORUS (mg)	TOTAL FAT (g)
atlantic, raw	100.0	g	82	17.8	0.0	54.00	412.9	202.9	0.67
	113.4	g	93	20.2	0.0	61.23	468.3	230.1	0.76
	4.00	oz							
atlantic, canned	100.0	g	105	22.8	0.0	218.0	528.0	260.0	0.86
	56.70	g	60	12.9	0.0	123.6	299.3	147.4	0.49
	2.00	oz							
atlantic, cooked, dry heat	100.0	g	105	22.8	0.0	78.00	244.0	138.0	0.86
	85.05	g	89	19.4	0.0	66.34	207.5	117.3	0.73
	3.00	oz							
pacific, raw	100.0	g	69	15.3	0.0	302.9	234.9	280.9	0.41
	113.4	g	78	17.3	0.0	343.5	266.4	318.6	0.46
	4.00	oz							
pacific, cooked, dry heat	100.0	g	85	18.7	0.0	372.0	289.0	345.0	0.50
	85.05	g	72	15.9	0.0	316.3	245.8	293.4	0.43
	3.00	oz							
ANCHOVIES									
Raw	100.0	g	131	20.4	0.0	104.0	382.9	173.9	4.84
	113.4	g	149	23.1	0.0	117.9	434.2	197.3	5.49
	4.00	oz							
canned, in oil, drained	100.0	g	210	28.9	0.0	3,668	544.0	252.0	9.71
	16.00	g	34	4.6	0.0	586.8	87.04	40.32	1.55
	4.00	pcs							
SHRIMP									
mixed species, raw	100.0	g	71	13.6	0.9	566.0	113.0	244.0	1.01
	113.4	g	81	15.4	1.0	641.8	128.1	276.4	1.15
	4.00	oz							
mixed species, breaded, fried	100.0	g	242	21.4	12	343.8	224.8	217.8	12.27
	85.05	g	206	18.2	9.8	292.4	191.2	185.3	10.44
	3.00	oz							
mixed species, cooked, moist heat	100.0	g	119	22.8	1.5	947.0	170.0	306.0	1.70
	85.05	g	101	19.4	1.3	805.4	144.5	260.2	1.45
	3.00	oz							
cracker	100.0	g	426	7.1	59	571.0	193.0	191.0	17.86

CLAMS

	SERVING QUANTITY	SERVING UNIT	CALORIES (KCal)	PROTEIN (g)	TOTAL CARBOHYDRATES (g)	SODIUM (mg)	POTASSIUM (mg)	PHOSPHORUS (mg)	TOTAL FAT (g)
mixed species, raw	100.0	g	86	14.7	3.6	601.0	46.00	198.0	0.96
	85.05	g	73	12.5	3.0	511.1	39.12	168.4	0.82
	3.00	oz							
mixed species, breaded, fried	100.0	g	202	14.2	10.3	364.0	326.0	188.0	11.15
	85.05	g	172	12.1	8.8	309.5	277.2	159.9	9.48
	3.00	oz							
mixed species, canned, with liquid	100.0	g	2	0.4	0.1	215.0	149.0	114.0	0.02
	28.35	g	1	0.1	0.0	60.95	42.24	32.32	0.01
	1.00	oz							
mixed species, canned, drained	100.0	g	142	24.3	5.9	112.0	628.0	327.0	1.59
	56.70	g	81	13.8	3.4	63.50	356.0	185.4	0.90
	2.00	oz							

OYSTERS

	SERVING QUANTITY	SERVING UNIT	CALORIES (KCal)	PROTEIN (g)	TOTAL CARBOHYDRATES (g)	SODIUM (mg)	POTASSIUM (mg)	PHOSPHORUS (mg)	TOTAL FAT (g)
ostrich, raw	100.0	g	125	21.6	0.0	83.00	297.0	204.0	3.67
	85.05	g	106	18.3	0.0	70.59	252.6	173.5	3.12
	3.00	oz							
ostrich, cooked	100.0	g	159	28.8	0.0	81.00	409.0	281.0	3.97
	85.05	g	135	24.5	0.0	68.89	347.8	239.0	3.38
	3.00	oz							
pacific, raw	100.0	g	81	9.5	5.0	106.0	168.0	162.0	2.30
	113.4	g	92	10.7	5.6	120.2	190.5	183.7	2.61
	4.00	oz							
pacific, cooked, moist heat	100.0	g	163	18.9	9.9	212.0	302.0	243.0	4.60
	85.05	g	139	16.1	8.4	180.3	256.8	206.6	3.91
	3.00	oz							
eastern, canned	100.0	g	68	7.1	3.9	112.0	229.0	139.0	2.47
	56.70	g	39	4.0	2.2	63.50	129.8	78.81	1.40
	2.00	oz							
eastern, farmed, raw	100.0	g	59	5.2	5.5	178.0	124.0	93.00	1.55
	85.05	g	50	4.4	4.7	151.4	105.4	79.10	1.32
	3.00	oz							
eastern, wild, raw	100.0	g	51	5.7	2.7	85.00	156.0	97.00	1.71
	113.4	g	58	6.5	3.1	96.39	176.9	110.0	1.94
	4.00	oz							
eastern, wild, breaded, fried	100.0	g	199	8.8	11.6	417.0	244.0	159.0	12.58
	85.05	g	169	7.5	9.9	354.6	207.5	135.2	10.70
	3.00	oz							
battered, breaded, fried, fast food	100.0	g	265	9.0	28.7	487.0	131.0	141.0	12.90
	85.05	g	225	7.7	24.4	414.1	111.4	119.9	10.97
	3.00	oz							

CRAB

	SERVING QUANTITY	SERVING UNIT	CALORIES (kCal)	PROTEIN (g)	TOTAL CARBOHYDRATES (g)	SODIUM (mg)	POTASSIUM (mg)	PHOSPHORUS (mg)	TOTAL FAT (g)
blue, raw	100.0	g	87	18.1	0.0	293.0	329.0	229.0	1.08
	113.4	g	99	20.5	0.5	332.2	373.1	259.7	1.22
	4.00	oz							
blue, canned	100.0	g	83	17.9	0.0	563.0	259.0	234.0	0.74
	56.70	g	47	10.1	0.0	319.2	146.8	132.6	0.42
	2.00	oz							
dungeness, raw	100.0	g	86	17.4	0.7	295.0	354.0	182.0	0.97
	113.4	g	98	19.7	0.8	334.5	401.4	206.4	1.10
	4.00	oz							
dungeness, cooked, moist heat	100.0	g	110	22.3	1.0	378.0	408.0	175.0	1.24
	85.05	g	94	19.0	0.8	321.5	347.0	148.8	1.05
	3.00	oz							
alaska king, raw	100.0	g	84	18.3	0.0	836.0	204.0	219.0	0.60
	113.4	g	95	20.7	0.0	948.0	231.3	248.3	0.68
	4.00	oz							
alaska king, cooked, moist heat	100.0	g	97	19.4	0.0	1,072	262.0	280.0	1.54
	85.05	g	83	16.5	0.0	911.7	222.8	238.1	1.31
	3.00	oz							
imitation, crabmeat (Kani)	100.0	g	95	7.6	15.0	529.0	90.00	282.0	0.46
	85.05	g	81	6.5	12.8	449.9	76.54	239.8	0.39
	3.00	oz							
cakes	100.0	g	266	18.8	8.5	819.0	270.0	378.0	17.25
	60.00	g	160	11.3	5.1	491.0	162.0	226.8	10.35
	1.00	pc							

CATFISH

	SERVING QUANTITY	SERVING UNIT	CALORIES (kCal)	PROTEIN (g)	TOTAL CARBOHYDRATES (g)	SODIUM (mg)	POTASSIUM (mg)	PHOSPHORUS (mg)	TOTAL FAT (g)
channel, wild, raw	100.0	g	95	16.4	0.0	43.00	405.9	208.9	2.82
	113.4	g	108	18.6	0.0	48.76	357.9	236.9	3.20
	4.00	oz							
channel, farmed, raw	100.0	g	119	15.2	0.0	97.94	301.8	203.8	5.94
	85.05	g	101	13.0	0.0	83.30	256.7	173.4	5.05
	3.00	oz							
breaded, fried	100.0	g	229	18.1	8.0	280.0	340.0	216.0	13.33
	85.05	g	195	15.4	6.8	238.1	289.1	183.7	11.34
	3.00	oz							
wild, cooked, dry heat	100.0	g	105	18.5	0.0	50.00	419.0	304.0	2.85
	85.05	g	89	15.7	0.0	42.52	356.3	258.5	2.42
	3.00	oz							
farmed, cooked, dry heat	100.0	g	144	18.4	0.0	119.0	366.0	247.0	7.19
	85.05	g	122	15.7	0.0	101.2	311.2	210.0	6.12
	3.00	oz							

	SERVING QUANTITY	SERVING UNIT	CALORIES (kCal)	PROTEIN (g)	TOTAL CARBOHYDRATES (g)	SODIUM (mg)	POTASSIUM (mg)	PHOSPHORUS (mg)	TOTAL FAT (g)
MUSSELS									
blue, raw	100.0	g	86	11.9	3.7	286.0	320.0	197.0	2.24
	113.4	g	98	13.5	4.2	324.3	362.8	223.4	2.54
	4.00	oz							
blue, cooked, moist heat	100.0	g	172	23.8	7.4	369.0	268.0	285.0	4.48
	85.05	g	146	20.2	6.3	313.8	227.9	242.4	3.81
	3.00	oz							
atlantic or pacific, meat only	100.0	g	197	8.8	11.6	415.2	243.8	159.0	12.56
	85.05	g	167	7.5	9.9	353.1	207.4	1,315	10.69
	3.00	oz							
MACKEREL									
Atlantic or Boston, raw fillet	100.0	g	205	18.6	0.0	89.99	313.9	216.9	13.89
	113.4	g	232	21.1	0.0	102.0	356.0	246.0	15.75
	4.00	oz							
pacific and Jack, raw fillet	100.0	g	158	20.1	0.0	85.99	405.9	125.0	7.89
	113.4	g	179	22.8	0.0	97.51	460.3	141.7	8.95
	4.00	oz							
Atlantic Spanish, raw fillet	100.0	g	139	19.3	0.0	58.99	445.9	204.9	6.30
	113.4	g	158	21.9	0.0	66.90	505.7	232.4	7.14
	4.00	oz							
Jack, canned, solids, drained	100.0	g	156	23.2	0.0	379.0	194.0	301.0	6.30
	56.70	g	88	13.2	0.0	214.8	110.0	170.6	3.57
	2.00	oz							
Atlantic or Boston, cooked, dry heat	100.0	g	262	23.9	0.0	83.00	401.0	278.0	17.81
	85.05	g	223	20.3	0.0	70.59	341.0	236.4	15.15
	3.00	oz							
Atlantic, Spanish, cooked, dry heat	100.0	g	158	23.6	0.0	66.00	554.0	271.0	6.32
	85.05	g	134	20.1	0.0	56.13	471.1	230.4	5.38
	3.00	oz							
Pacific and Jack, mixed species, cooked	100.0	g	201	25.7	0.0	110.0	521.0	160.0	10.12
	85.05	g	171	21.9	0.0	93.55	443.1	136.0	8.61
	3.00	oz							

TROUT	SERVING QUANTITY	SERVING UNIT	CALORIES (kCal)	PROTEIN (g)	TOTAL CARBOHYDRATES (g)	SODIUM (mg)	POTASSIUM (mg)	PHOSPHORUS (mg)	TOTAL FAT (g)
rainbow, wild, raw, fillet	100.0	g	119	20.5	0.0	31.00	481.0	271.0	3.46
	113.4	g	135	23.2	0.0	35.15	545.4	307.3	3.92
	4.00	oz							
rainbow, farmed, raw, fillet	100.0	g	141	19.9	0.0	51.00	376.9	225.9	6.18
	113.4	g	160	22.6	0.0	57.83	427.4	256.2	7.01
	4.00	oz							
mixed species, raw fillet	100.0	g	148	20.8	0.0	52.00	360.9	244.9	6.61
	113.4	g	168	23.6	0.0	58.96	409.3	277.8	7.50
	4.00	oz							
sea trout, mixed species, raw	100.0	g	104	16.7	0.0	57.99	340.9	249.9	3.61
	113.4	g	118	19.0	0.0	65.77	386.6	283.4	4.09
	4.00	oz							
rainbow, wild, cooked, dry heat	100.0	g	150	22.9	0.0	56.00	448.0	269.0	5.82
	85.05	g	128	19.5	0.0	47.63	381.0	228.7	4.95
	3.00	oz							
rainbow, farmed, cooked, dry heat	100.0	g	168	23.8	0.0	61.00	450.0	270.0	7.38
	85.05	g	143	20.2	0.0	51.88	382.7	229.6	6.28
	3.00	oz							
mixed species, cooked, dry heat	100.0	g	190	26.6	0.0	67.00	463.0	314.0	8.47
	85.05	g	162	22.7	0.0	56.98	393.7	267.0	7.20
	3.00	oz							
sea trout, mixed species, cooked, dry heat	100.0	g	133	21.5	0.0	74.00	437.0	321.0	4.63
	85.05	g	113	18.3	0.0	62.94	371.6	273.0	3.94
	3.00	oz							
CARP									
raw	100.0	g	127	17.8	0.0	49.00	332.9	414.9	5.60
	113.4	g	144	20.2	0.0	55.56	377.6	470.5	6.35
	4.00	oz							
cooked, dry heat	100.0	g	162	22.9	0.0	63.00	427.0	531.0	7.17
	85.05	g	138	19.4	0.0	53.58	363.1	451.6	6.10
	3.00	oz							
MAHI-MAHI									
Dorado or Dolphinfish, raw	100.0	g	85	18.5	0.0	87.99	415.9	143.0	0.70
	113.4	g	96	21.0	0.0	99.78	471.7	162.1	0.79
	4.00	oz							
Doradao or Dolphinfish, cooked, dry heat	100.0	g	109	23.7	0.0	113.0	533.0	183.0	0.90
	85.05	g	93	20.2	0.0	96.11	452.3	155.6	0.77
	3.00	oz							

	SERVING QUANTITY	SERVING UNIT	CALORIES (kCal)	PROTEIN (g)	TOTAL CARBOHYDRATES (g)	SODIUM (mg)	POTASSIUM (mg)	PHOSPHORUS (mg)	TOTAL FAT (g)
FLATFISH									
raw	100.0	g	70	12.4	0.0	295.9	159.9	251.9	1.93
	113.4	g	79	14.1	0.0	335.6	181.4	285.7	2.19
	4.00	oz							
cooked, dry heat	100.0	g	86	15.2	0.0	363.0	197.0	309.0	2.37
	85.05	g	73	13.0	0.0	308.7	167.5	262.8	2.02
	3.00	oz							
HALIBUT									
greenland, raw	100.0	g	186	14.4	0.0	80.0	267.9	163.9	13.84
	113.4	g	211	16.3	0.0	90.7	303.8	185.9	15.69
	4.00	oz							
atlantic and pacific, raw	100.0	g	91	18.6	0.0	68.0	434.9	235.9	1.33
	113.4	g	103	21.0	0.0	77.10	493.2	267.6	1.51
	4.00	oz							
greenland, cooked, dry heat	100.0	g	239	18.4	0.0	103.0	344.0	210.0	17.71
	85.05	g	203	15.7	0.0	87.60	292.5	178.6	15.09
	3.00	oz							
atlantic and pacific, cooked, dry heat	100.0	g	111	22.5	0.0	82.00	528.0	287.0	1.61
	85.05	g	94	19.2	0.0	69.74	449.0	244.1	1.37
	3.00	oz							
LOBSTER									
Northern, raw (Langoustine)	100.0	g	77	16.5	0.0	423.0	200.0	161.0	0.75
	113.4	g	87	18.7	0.0	479.6	226.8	182.5	0.85
	4.00	oz							
Spiny, mixed species, raw	100.0	g	112	20.6	2.4	177.0	180.0	238.0	1.51
	113.4	g	127	23.4	2.8	200.7	104.1	269.9	1.71
	4.00	oz							
Northern, cooked, moist heat (Langoustine)	100.0	g	89	19.0	0.0	486.0	230.0	185.0	0.86
	85.05	g	76	16.2	0.0	413.3	195.6	157.3	0.73
	3.00	oz							
Spiny, mixed species, cooked, moist heat	100.0	g	143	26.4	3.1	227.0	208.0	229.0	1.94
	85.05	g	122	22.5	2.7	193.0	176.9	194.7	1.65
	3.00	oz							

SCALLOPS	SERVING QUANTITY	SERVING UNIT	CALORIES (kCal)	PROTEIN (g)	TOTAL CARBOHYDRATES (g)	SODIUM (mg)	POTASSIUM (mg)	PHOSPHORUS (mg)	TOTAL FAT (g)
Mixed species, raw	100.0	g	69	12.1	3.2	392.0	205.0	12.80	0.49
	113.4	g	78	13.7	3.6	444.5	232.4	14.52	0.56
	4.00	oz							
Bay and Sea, steamed	100.0	g	111	20.5	5.4	667.0	314.0	426.0	0.84
	85.05	g	94	17.5	4.6	567.2	267.0	362.3	0.71
	3.00	oz							
mixed species, breaded and fried	100.0	g	216	18.1	10.1	464.0	333.0	236.0	10.94
	46.50	g	100	8.4	4.7	215.7	15.85	109.7	5.09
	3.00	pcs							
breaded, fried, fast food	100.0	g	268	10.9	26.7	638.0	204.0	203.0	13.47
	85.05	g	228	9.3	22.7	542.6	173.5	172.6	11.46
	3.00	oz							
HERRING									
Pacific, raw	100.0	g	195	16.4	0.0	73.99	422.9	227.9	13.88
	113.4	g	221	18.6	0.0	83.91	479.6	258.5	15.74
	4.00	oz							
Atlantic, raw	100.0	g	158	18.0	0.0	89.99	326.9	235.9	9.04
	113.4	g	179	20.4	0.0	102.0	370.7	267.6	10.25
	4.00	oz							
Pacific, cooked, dry heat	100.0	g	250	21.0	0.0	95.00	542.0	292.0	17.79
	85.05	g	213	17.9	0.0	80.80	460.9	248.3	15.13
	3.00	oz							
Atlantic, cooked, dry heat	100.0	g	203	23.0	0.0	115.0	419.0	303.0	11.49
	85.05	g	173	19.6	0.0	97.81	356.3	257.7	9.86
	3.00	oz							
Roe or eggs, Pacific (Alaska Native)	100.0	g	74	9.6	4.5	61.00	na	na	1.93
	85.05	g	63	8.2	3.8	51.88	na	na	1.64
	3.00	oz							

CRAYFISH/ CRAWFISH	SERVING QUANTITY	SERVING UNIT	CALORIES (kCal)	PROTEIN (g)	TOTAL CARBOHYDRATES (g)	SODIUM (mg)	POTASSIUM (mg)	PHOSPHORUS (mg)	TOTAL FAT (g)
Mixed species, farmed, raw	100.0	g	72	14.9	0.0	62.00	261.0	218.0	0.97
	113.4 4.00	g oz	82	16.8	0.0	70.31	295.9	247.2	1.10
Mixed species, wild, raw	100.0	g	77	16.0	0.0	58.00	302.0	256.0	0.95
	113.4 4.00	g oz	87	18.1	0.0	65.77	342.4	290.3	1.08
Mixed species, farmed, cooked, moist heat	100.0	g	87	17.5	0.0	97.00	238.0	241.0	0.22
	85.05 3.00	g oz	74	14.9	0.0	82.50	202.4	204.9	0.18
mixed species, wild, cooked, moist heat	100.0	g	82	16.8	0.0	94.00	296.0	270.0	1.20
	85.05 3.00	g oz	70	14.3	0.0	79.95	251.7	229.6	1.02
SQUID (CALAMARI)									
mixed species, fried	100.0	g	175	17.9	7.8	306.0	279.0	251.0	7.48
	85.05 3.00	g oz	149	15.3	6.6	260.3	237.3	213.4	6.36
mixed species, raw	100.0	g	92	15.6	3.1	44.00	246.0	221.0	1.38
boneless	113.4 4.00	g oz	104	17.7	3.5	49.90	278.9	250.6	1.56

EGG

	SERVING QUANTITY	SERVING UNIT	CALORIES (kCal)	PROTEIN (g)	TOTAL CARBOHYDRATES (g)	SODIUM (mg)	POTASSIUM (mg)	PHOSPHORUS (mg)	TOTAL FAT (g)
chicken, raw, large	100.0	g	143	12.6	0.7	142.0	138.0	198.0	9.51
	50.00	g	72	6.3	0.4	71.00	69.00	99.00	4.76
	1.00	pc							
chicken, fried, large	100.0	g	196	13.6	0.8	207.0	152.0	215.0	14.84
	46.00	g	90	6.3	0.4	95.22	69.92	98.90	6.83
	1.00	pc							
chicken, poached, large	100.0	g	143	12.5	0.7	297.0	138.0	197.0	9.47
	50.00	g	72	6.3	0.4	148.5	69.00	98.50	4.74
	1.00	pc							
chicken, hard boiled, large	100.0	g	155	12.6	1.1	124.0	126.0	172.0	10.61
	50.00	g	78	6.3	0.6	62.00	63.00	86.00	5.31
	1.00	pc							
scrambled, fast food	100.0	g	212	13.8	2.1	187.0	147.0	242.0	16.18
	94.00	g	199	13.0	2.0	175.7	138.1	227.4	15.21
	2.00	pc							
substitute, liquid	100.0	g	84	12.0	0.6	177.0	330.0	121.0	3.31
	251.0	g	211	30.1	1.6	444.2	828.3	303.7	8.31
	1.00	c							
substitute, powder	100.0	g	443	55.8	22	798.2	742.3	476.9	12.97
	9.92	g	44	5.5	2.2	79.20	73.66	47.32	1.29
	0.35	oz							
substitute, frozen	100.0	g	160	11.3	3.2	199.0	213.0	72.00	11.11
	60.00	g	96	6.8	1.9	119.4	127.8	43.20	6.67
	0.25	c							
chicken, egg whites only, raw large egg	100.0	g	52	10.9	0.7	166.0	163.0	15.00	0.17
	33.00	g	17	3.6	0.2	54.78	53.79	4.95	0.06
	1.00	pc							
chicken, yolk only, raw large egg	100.0	g	322	15.9	3.6	48.00	109.0	390.0	26.54
	17.00	g	55	2.7	0.6	8.16	18.53	66.30	4.51
	1.00	pc							
chicken, whole, raw, frozen	100.0	g	147	12.3	1.0	128.0	135.0	193.0	9.95
	56.70	g	83	7.0	0.6	72.57	76.54	109.4	5.64
	2.00	oz							
yolk only, frozen, raw	100.0	g	296	15.5	0.8	67.00	121.0	420.0	25.60
	56.70	g	168	8.8	0.5	37.99	68.61	238.1	14.51
	2.00	oz							
whites, frozen, raw	100.0	g	48	10.2	1.0	169.0	169.0	13.00	0.00
	56.70	g	27	5.8	0.6	95.82	95.82	7.37	0.00
	2.00	oz							
duck, raw	100.0	g	185	12.8	1.5	146.0	222.0	220.0	13.77
	70.00	g	130	9.0	1.0	102.2	155.4	154.0	9.64
	1.00	pc							
quail, raw	100.0	g	158	13.1	0.4	141.0	132.0	226.0	11.09
	9.00	g	14	1.2	0.0	12.69	11.88	20.34	1.00
	1.00	pc							

CHICKEN	SERVING QUANTITY	SERVING UNIT	CALORIES (kCal)	PROTEIN (g)	TOTAL CARBOHYDRATES (g)	SODIUM (mg)	POTASSIUM (mg)	PHOSPHORUS (mg)	TOTAL FAT (g)
ground, raw	100.0	g	143	17.4	0.0	60.00	522.0	178.0	8.10
meat and skin,	100.0	g	215	18.6	0.0	70.00	189.0	147.0	15.06
raw	113.4	g	244	21.1	0.0	79.38	214.3	166.7	17.08
	4.00	oz							
meat and skin,	100.0	g	239	27.3	0.0	82.00	223.0	182.0	13.60
roasted	85.05	g	203	23.2	0.0	69.74	189.6	154.8	11.57
	3.00	oz							
thigh meat	100.0	g	218	28.2	1.2	95.00	259.0	199.0	10.30
only, fried	85.05	g	185	24.0	1.0	80.80	220.2	169.2	8.76
	3.00	oz							
thigh meat	100.0	g	179	24.8	0.0	106.0	269.0	230.0	8.15
only, roasted	85.05	g	152	21.1	0.0	90.15	228.7	195.6	6.93
	3.00	oz							
wing meat	100.0	g	211	30.2	0.0	91.00	208.0	164.0	9.15
only, fried	85.05	g	179	25.6	0.0	77.39	176.9	139.4	7.78
	3.00	oz							
wing meat	100.0	g	203	30.5	0.0	92.00	210.0	166.0	8.13
only, roasted	85.05	g	173	26.0	0.0	78.25	178.6	141.1	6.91
	3.00	oz							
wing meat	100.0	g	181	27.2	0.0	73.00	153.0	134.0	7.18
only, stewed	85.05	g	154	23.1	0.0	62.09	130.1	113.9	6.11
	3.00	oz							
back meat	100.0	g	288	30.0	5.7	99.00	251.0	176.0	4.12
only, fried	85.05	g	245	25.5	4.8	84.20	213.4	149.7	3.50
	3.00	oz							
back meat	100.0	g	239	28.2	0.0	96.00	237.0	165.0	13.16
only, roasted	85.05	g	203	24.0	0.0	81.65	201.5	140.3	11.19
	3.00	oz							
back meat	100.0	g	209	25.3	0.0	67.00	158.0	130.0	11.19
only, stewed	85.05	g	178	21.5	0.0	56.98	134.3	110.5	9.52
	3.00	oz							
drumstick	100.0	g	195	28.6	0.0	96.00	249.0	186.0	8.08
meat only, fried	85.05	g	166	24.3	0.0	81.65	211.7	158.2	6.87
	3.00	oz							
drumstick	100.0	g	155	24.2	0.0	128.0	256.0	200.0	5.70
meat only, roasted	85.05	g	132	20.6	0.0	108.8	217.7	170.1	4.85
	3	oz							

CHICKEN	SERVING QUANTITY	SERVING UNIT	CALORIES (kCal)	PROTEIN (g)	TOTAL CARBOHYDRATES (g)	SODIUM (mg)	POTASSIUM (mg)	PHOSPHORUS (mg)	TOTAL FAT (g)
drumstick meat only, stewed	100.0	g	169	27.5	0.0	80.00	199.0	150.0	5.71
	85.05 3.00	g oz	144	23.4	0.0	68.04	169.2	127.5	4.86
leg meat only, fried	100.0	g	208	28.4	0.7	96.00	254.0	193.0	9.32
	85.05 3.00	g oz	177	24.1	0.6	81.65	216.0	164.1	7.93
leg meat only, roasted	100.0	g	174	24.2	0.0	99.00	269.0	205.0	7.80
	85.05 3.00	g oz	148	20.6	0.0	84.20	228.7	174.3	6.63
leg meat only, stewed	100.0	g	185	26.3	0.0	78.00	190.0	149.0	8.06
	85.05 3.00	g oz	157	22.3	0.0	66.34	161.6	126.7	6.85
pate, chicken liver, canned	100.0	g	201	13.5	6.6	386.0	95.00	175.0	13.10
	52.00 4.00	g tbsp	105	7.0	3.4	200.7	49.40	91.00	6.81
chicken tenders, fast food	100.0	g	271	19.2	17.3	769.0	373.0	282.0	13.95
	62.00 4.00	g pcs	168	11.9	10.7	476.8	231.2	174.8	8.65
chicken patty, frozen, cooked	100.0	g	287	14.9	12.8	532.0	261.0	208.0	19.58
bratwurst, chicken, cooked	100.0	g	176	19.4	0.0	72.00	211.0	160.0	10.30
	83.92 2.96	g oz	148	16.3	0.0	60.42	177.0	134.2	8.69
sausage, chicken/beef, smoked	100.0	g	295	18.5	0.0	1,020	139.0	111.0	244.0
	138.0 1.00	g c	251	15.7	0.0	867.5	118.2	94.41	20.41

TURKEY	SERVING QUANTITY	SERVING UNIT	CALORIES (kCal)	PROTEIN (g)	TOTAL CARBOHYDRATES (g)	SODIUM (mg)	POTASSIUM (mg)	PHOSPHORUS (mg)	TOTAL FAT (g)
breast, meat & skin, raw	100.0	g	144	21.6	0.1	112.0	224.0	183.0	5.64
	113.4	g	163	24.5	0.2	127.0	254.0	207.5	6.40
	4.00	oz							
breast, meat & skin, roasted	100.0	g	189	28.6	0.1	103.0	239.0	223.0	7.39
	85.05	g	161	24.3	0.1	87.60	203.2	189.6	6.29
	3.00	oz							
breast, meat only, raw	100.0	g	114	23.3	0.0	74.00	267.0	185.0	2.33
	85.05	g	97	19.9	0.0	62.94	227.0	157.3	1.98
	3.00	oz							
breast, meat only, roasted	100.0	g	136	29.5	0.0	114.0	297.0	253.0	1.97
	85.05	g	116	25.1	0.0	96.96	252.6	215.1	1.68
	3.00	oz							
ground, raw	100.0	g	148	20.0	0.0	58.00	237.0	200.0	7.66
	113.4	g	168	22.3	0.0	65.77	268.7	226.8	8.69
	4.00	oz							
ground, cooked	100.0	g	203	27.4	0.0	78.00	294.0	254.0	10.40
	85.05	g	173	23.3	0.0	66.34	250.0	216.0	8.85
	3.00	oz							
white rotisserie, deli cut	100.0	g	112	13.5	7.7	1,200	349.0	158.0	3.00
	56.70	g	64	7.7	4.4	680.4	197.8	89.59	1.70
	2.00	oz							
ham, extra lean, sliced	100.0	g	134	19.6	0.9	1,038	299.0	304.0	5.80
	20.00	g	27	3.9	0.2	207.6	59.80	60.80	1.16
	1.00	pc							
pastrami, sliced	100.0	g	139	16.3	3.3	1,123	345.0	200.0	6.21
	56.70	g	79	9.2	1.9	636.7	195.6	113.4	3.52
	2.00	slices							
bologna	100.0	g	209	11.4	4.7	1,071	135.0	114.0	16.05
	56.70	g	119	6.5	2.7	607.2	76.55	64.64	9.10
	2.00	slices							
salami	100.0	g	172	19.2	1.6	1,107	216.0	266.0	9.21
	56.70	g	98	10.9	0.9	627.6	122.4	150.8	5.22
	2.00	slices							
bacon, turkey, cooked	100.0	g	382	29.6	3.1	2,285	395.0	460.0	27.90
	28.35	g	108	8.4	0.9	647.8	111.9	130.4	7.91
	1.00	oz							
bacon, turkey, low sodium	100.0	g	253	13.3	4.8	900.0	156.0	145.0	20.00
	15.00	g	38	2.0	0.7	135.0	23.40	21.75	3.00
	1.00	svg							
sausage, turkey, cooked	100.0	g	196	23.9	0.0	665.0	298.0	202.0	10.44
	56.70	g	111	13.6	0.0	377.0	168.9	114.5	5.92
	2.00	oz							

PORK	SERVING QUANTITY	SERVING UNIT	CALORIES (kCal)	PROTEIN (g)	TOTAL CARBOHYDRATES (g)	SODIUM (mg)	POTASSIUM (mg)	PHOSPHORUS (mg)	TOTAL FAT (g)
ground, cooked	100.0	g	297	25.7	0.0	73.00	362.0	226.0	20.77
	85.05	g	253	21.9	0.0	62.09	307.8	192.2	17.66
	3.00	oz							
ground, raw	100.0	g	263	16.9	0.0	56.00	287.0	175.0	21.19
	113.4	g	298	19.1	0.0	63.50	325.4	198.4	24.03
	4.00	oz							
loin, sirloin, roasts, separable lean roasted	100.0	g	204	27.8	0.0	59.00	352.0	235.0	9.44
	85.05	g	174	23.6	0.0	50.18	299.3	199.8	8.03
	3.00	oz							
loin, center rib, separable lean, roasted	100.0	g	206	28.8	0.0	95.00	287.0	244.0	9.21
	85.05	g	175	24.5	0.0	80.80	244.1	207.5	7.83
	3.00	oz							
loin, sirloin, boneless, separable lean roasted	100.0	g	178	30.4	0.0	66.00	408.0	311.0	5.31
	85.05	g	151	25.9	0.0	56.13	347.0	264.5	4.52
	3.00	oz							
loin, center rib, boneless roasted	100.0	g	214	28.8	0.0	50.00	363.0	222.0	10.13
	85.05	g	182	24.5	0.0	42.52	308.7	188.8	8.62
	3.00	oz							
shoulder blade, boston roasts roasted	100.0	g	232	24.2	0.0	88.00	427.0	235.0	14.30
	85.05	g	197	20.6	0.0	74.84	363.1	199.8	12.16
	3.00	oz							
turkey, salt. shoulder, whole, roasted	100.0	g	230	25.3	0.0	74.96	345.8	220.8	13.53
	85.05	g	196	21.5	0.0	63.75	294.1	187.8	11.51
	3.00	oz							
loin, whole, roasted	100.0	g	209	28.6	0.0	58.00	425.0	249.0	9.63
	85.05	g	178	24.3	0.0	49.33	361.4	211.7	8.19
	3.00	oz							
leg or ham, whole, roasted	100.0	g	211	29.4	0.0	64.00	373.0	281.0	9.44
	85.05	g	179	25.0	0.0	54.43	317.2	239.0	8.03
	3.00	oz							
loin, tenderloin, separable lean & fat roasted	100.0	g	147	26.0	0.0	57.00	419.0	265.0	3.96
	85.05	g	125	22.2	0.0	48.48	356.3	225.3	3.37
	3.00	oz							
ground, cooked	100.0	g	297	25.7	0.0	73.00	362.0	226.0	20.77
	85.05	g	253	21.9	0.0	62.09	307.8	192.2	17.66
	3.00	oz							

PORK

PORK	SERVING QUANTITY	SERVING UNIT	CALORIES (KCal)	PROTEIN (g)	TOTAL CARBOHYDRATES (g)	SODIUM (mg)	POTASSIUM (mg)	PHOSPHORUS (mg)	TOTAL FAT (g)
bacon, cured, broiled, panfried or roasted	100.0	g	541	37.0	1.4	1,717	565.0	533.0	41.78
	8.00	g	43	3.0	0.1	137.3	45.20	42.64	3.34
	1.00	slice							
bacon, reduced sodium, cured broiled, panfried or roasted	100.0	g	541	37.0	1.4	1,030	565.0	533.0	41.78
	56.70	g	307	21.0	0.8	584.0	320.4	302.2	23.69
	2.00	oz							
country style ribs, separable lean & fat roasted	100.0	g	359	21.8	0.0	52.00	322.0	214.0	29.46
	85.05	g	305	18.5	0.0	44.23	273.9	182.0	25.06
	3.00	oz							
sirloin, chops or roasts, boneless, raw	100.0	g	121	22.8	0.0	63.00	354.0	251.0	2.59
	113.4	g	137	25.9	0.0	71.44	401.4	284.6	2.94
	4.00	oz							
kidney, braised	100.0	g	151	25.4	0.0	80.00	143.0	240.0	4.70
	85.05	g	128	21.6	0.0	68.04	121.6	204.1	4.00
	3.00	oz							
liver, braised	100.0	g	165	26.0	3.8	49.00	150.0	241.0	4.40
	85.05	g	140	22.1	3.2	41.67	127.6	205.0	3.74
	3.00	oz							
ham, minced, sliced	100.0	g	263	16.3	1.8	1,245	311.0	157.0	20.68
	21.00	g	55	3.4	0.4	261.4	65.31	32.97	4.34
	1.00	slice							
ham, extra lean, 5% fat	100.0	g	107	16.9	0.7	945.0	463.0	252.0	4.04
	85.05	g	91	14.3	0.6	803.7	393.8	214.3	3.44
	3.00	oz							
ham, low sodium, cured, cooked	100.0	g	165	22.0	0.5	969.0	362.0	248.0	7.70
	85.05	g	140	18.7	0.4	824.1	307.9	210.9	6.55
	3.00	oz							
sausages, Kielbasa, grilled	100.0	g	337	12.5	5.0	1,062	306.0	204.0	29.68
	85.05	g	287	10.6	4.3	903.2	260.3	173.5	25.24
	3.00	oz							
Kielbasa, panfried	100.0	g	333	12.4	4.8	1,046	304.0	199.0	29.43
	85.05	g	283	10.5	4.1	889.6	258.6	169.3	25.03
	3.00	oz							
Beerwurst, pork/beef	100.0	g	276	14.0	4.3	732.0	244.0	135.0	22.53
	56.70	g	156	7.9	2.4	415.0	138.4	76.6	12.77
	2.00	oz							

PORK	SERVING QUANTITY	SERVING UNIT	CALORIES (kCal)	PROTEIN (g)	TOTAL CARBOHYDRATES	SODIUM (mg)	POTASSIUM (mg)	PHOSPHORUS (mg)	TOTAL FAT (g)
Italian Sweet, links	100.0	g	149	16.1	2.1	570.0	194.0	103.0	8.42
	85.05 3	g oz	127	13.7	1.8	484.8	165.0	87.60	7.16
Polish, pork, cooked	100.0	g	326	14.1	1.6	876.0	237.0	136.0	28.72
	56.70 2	g oz	185	8.0	0.9	496.6	134.3	77.11	16.28
Bratwurst, pork, cooked	100.0	g	333	13.7	2.9	846.0	348.0	208.0	29.18
	56.70 2	g oz	189	7.8	1.6	479.6	197.3	117.9	16.54
meatloaf/ luncheon meat pork/beef	100.0	g	260	15.4	1.6	1,182	245.0	122.0	20.90
	2.0 1	g slice	60	3.5	0.4	271.8	56.35	28.06	4.81
peperoni, beef/pork	100.0	g	504	19.3	1.2	1,582	274.0	158.0	46.28
	56.70 2	g oz	286	11.0	0.7	896.9	155.3	89.58	26.24
salami, italian, pork	100.0	g	425	21.7	1.2	1,890	340.0	229.0	37.00
	28.35 1	g oz	120	6.2	0.3	535.8	96.39	64.92	10.49

BEEF

BEEF	SERVING QUANTITY	SERVING UNIT	CALORIES (kCal)	PROTEIN (g)	TOTAL CARBOHYDRATES (g)	SODIUM (mg)	POTASSIUM (mg)	PHOSPHORUS (mg)	TOTAL FAT (g)
chuck eyeroast, boneless, all grades 0" fat, separable lean only, ***roasted***	3.0	g	183	26.7	0.0	68.04	344.0	210.0	8.46
	85.05	g	156	22.7	0.0	80.00	292.5	178.6	7.20
	3.00	oz							
chuck eyeroast, boneless, all grades separable lean only, 0", ***raw***	100.0	g	137	20.6	0.0	85.00	357.0	204.0	6.01
	85.05	g	117	17.5	0.0	72.29	303.6	173.5	5.11
	3.00	oz							
chuck eyeroast, boneless, all grades sep lean & fat, 0" fat, ***roasted***	100.0	g	236	24.6	0.0	76.00	308.0	187.0	15.29
	85.05	g	201	21.0	0.0	64.64	261.9	159.0	13.00
	3.00	oz							
chuck eyeroast, boneless, all grades sep lean & fat, 0" fat, ***raw***	100.0	g	173	19.3	0.0	82.00	367.0	187.0	10.67
	85.05	g	147	16.4	0.0	69.74	312.1	159.0	9.07
	3.00	oz							
jerky	100.0	g	410	33.2	11	1,785	597.0	407.0	25.60
	28.35	g	116	9.4	3.1	506.0	169.2	115.3	7.26
	1.00	oz							
corned beef, brisket, ***raw***	100.0	g	198	14.7	0.1	1,217	297.0	117.0	14.90
	113.4	g	225	16.7	0.2	1,380	336.8	132.6	16.90
	4.00	oz							
corned beef, brisket, ***cooked***	100.0	g	251	18.2	0.5	928.0	145.0	125.0	18.98
	85.05	g	213	15.5	0.4	827.5	123.3	106.3	16.14
	3.00	oz							
broth cube 1 cube, 6 fl. oz prepared	100.0	g	170	17.3	16	24,000	403.0	225.0	4.00
	3.60	g	6	0.6	0.6	864.0	14.51	8.10	0.14
	1.00	cube							
liver, pan fried	100.0	g	175	26.5	5.2	77.00	351.0	485.0	4.68
	81.00	g	142	21.5	4.2	62.37	284.3	392.8	3.79
	1.00	slice							
liver, braised	100.0	g	191	29.1	5.1	79.00	352.0	497.0	5.26
	85.05	g	162	24.7	4.4	67.19	299.3	422.7	4.47
	3.00	oz							
tongue, simmered	100.0	g	284	19.3	0.0	65.00	184.0	145.0	22.30
	85.05	g	242	16.4	0.0	55.28	156.5	123.3	18.97
	3.00	oz							
kidney simmered	100.0	g	158	27.3	0.0	94.00	135.0	304.0	4.65
	85.05	g	134	23.2	0.0	79.95	114.8	258.5	3.95
	3.00	oz							
tripe, simmered	100.0	g	94	11.7	2.0	68.00	42.00	66.00	4.05
	85.05	g	80	10.0	1.7	57.83	35.72	56.13	3.44
	3.00	oz							

LAMB

	SERVING QUANTITY	SERVING UNIT	CALORIES (kCal)	PROTEIN (g)	TOTAL CARBOHYDRATES (g)	SODIUM (mg)	POTASSIUM (mg)	PHOSPHORUS (mg)	TOTAL FAT (g)
tenderloin, New Zealand, separable lean only, **raw**	100.0	g	116	20.5	0.0	49.00	381.0	222.0	3.81
	85.05	g	99	17.5	0.0	41.67	324.0	188.8	3.24
	3.00	oz							
loin, NZ, separable lean, frozen, **broiled**	100.0	g	199	29.3	0.0	55.00	189.0	240.0	8.24
	85.05	g	169	24.9	0.0	46.78	160.7	204.1	7.01
	3.00	oz							
australian, separable lean, 1/8" fat, **cooked**	100.0	g	201	26.7	0.0	80.00	318.0	207.0	9.63
	85.05	g	171	22.7	0.0	68.04	270.4	176.0	8.19
	3.00	oz							
Australian, separable lean, 1/8" fat, **raw**	100.0	g	142	20.3	0.0	83.00	320.0	188.0	6.18
	113.4	g	161	23.0	0.0	94.12	362.8	213.2	7.01
	4.00	oz							
Australian, ground, 85%Lean/15%fat, **raw**	100.0	g	255	17.1	0.0	65.49	Na	Na	20.17
	85.05	g	217	14.6	0.0	77.00	Na	Na	17.61
	3.00	oz							
NZ, rib, separable lean, frozen, **raw**	100.0	g	160	20.7	0.0	67.00	309.0	185.0	8.61
	113.4	g	181	23.4	0.0	75.98	350.4	209.8	9.76
	4.00	oz							
NZ, rib, separable lean, frozen, **roasted**	100.0	g	193	24.4	0.0	72.00	323.0	209.0	10.63
	85.05	g	164	20.8	0.0	61.24	274.7	177.7	9.04
	3.00	oz							

VEAL

	SERVING QUANTITY	SERVING UNIT	CALORIES (kCal)	PROTEIN (g)	TOTAL CARBOHYDRATES (g)	SODIUM (mg)	POTASSIUM (mg)	PHOSPHORUS (mg)	TOTAL FAT (g)
separable lean, cooked	100.0	g	196	32.0	0.0	89.00	338.0	250.0	6.58
	85.05	g	167	27.1	0.0	75.69	287.4	212.6	5.60
	3.00	oz							
	100.0	g	193	27.4	4.5	85.00	353.0	483.0	6.51
liver, pan fried	85.05	g	164	23.3	3.8	72.29	300.2	410.8	5.54
	3.00	oz							
sausage, bratwurst, veal, cooked	100.0	g	341	14.0	0.0	60.00	231.0	150.0	31.70
	83.92	g	286	11.7	0.0	50.35	193.8	125.8	26.60
	2.96	oz							
ground, pan fried	100.0	g	503	8.9	0.9	89.00	107.0	133.0	51.60
	85.05	g	428	7.5	0.8	75.69	91.00	113.1	43.89
	3.00	oz							

VEAL	SERVING QUANTITY	SERVING UNIT	CALORIES (kCal)	PROTEIN (g)	TOTAL CARBOHYDRATES (g)	SODIUM (mg)	POTASSIUM (mg)	PHOSPHORUS (mg)	TOTAL FAT (g)
sirloin, separable, lean, braised	100.0	g	204	34.0	0.0	81.00	339.0	259.0	6.51
	85.05	g	174	28.9	0.0	68.89	288.3	220.2	5.54
	3.00	oz							
sirloin separable lean, roasted	100.0	g	168	26.3	0.0	85.00	365.0	231.0	6.22
	85.05	g	143	22.4	0.0	72.29	310.4	196.4	5.29
	3.00	oz							
sirloin, lean, raw	100.0	g	110	20.2	0.0	80.00	348.0	220.0	2.59
	113.4	g	125	22.9	0.0	90.72	394.6	249.4	2.94
	4.00	oz							
loin, lean and fat, braised	100.0	g	284	30.2	0.0	80.00	280.0	220.0	17.21
	85.05	g	242	25.7	0.0	68.04	238.1	187.1	14.64
	3.00	oz							
loin, lean and fat, roasted	100.0	g	217	25.0	0.0	93.00	325.0	212.0	12.32
	85.05	g	185	21.1	0.0	79.10	276.4	180.3	10.48
	3.00	oz							
loin, lean, braised	100.0	g	226	33.6	0.0	84.00	297.0	237.0	9.15
	85.05	g	192	28.6	0.0	71.44	252.6	201.5	7.78
	3.00	oz							
loin, lean, roasted	100.0	g	175	26.3	0.0	96.00	340.0	222.0	6.94
	85.05	g	149	22.4	0.0	81.65	289.1	188.8	5.90
	3.00	oz							
loin, lean, raw	100.0	g	114	21.9	0.0	99.00	260.0	237.0	2.90
	113.4	g	129	24.8	0.0	112.2	294.8	268.7	3.29
	4.00	oz							
loin, chop, lean and fat, grilled	100.0	g	198	28.0	0.2	86.00	229.0	208.0	9.48
	85.05	g	168	23.9	0.1	73.14	194.7	176.9	8.06
	3.00	oz							
bratwwurst, veal, cooked	100.0	g	341	14.0	0.0	60.00	231.0	150.0	31.70
	83.92	g	286	11.7	0.0	50.35	193.8	125.8	26.60
	2.96	oz							

H. Herbs and Spices

Hey there!

Do you need to print out this Food List?

You can download a printable version of this chart by scanning the QR code below or copying the link on your computer browser.

https://go.renaltracker.com/printfoodlist

	SERVING QUANTITY	SERVING UNIT	CALORIES (kCal)	PROTEIN (g)	TOTAL CARBOHYDRATES (g)	SODIUM (mg)	POTASSIUM (mg)	PHOSPHORUS (mg)	TOTAL FAT (g)
ONION									
red, raw	100.0	g	44	0.94	9.93	1	197	41	0.1
1 onion	197.0	g	86.7	1.85	19.6	1.97	388	80.8	0.19
white, raw	100.0	g	36	0.89	7.68	2	141	29	0.13
yellow, raw	100.0	g	38	0.83	8.61	1	182	34	0.05
1 onion	143.0	g	54.3	1.19	12.3	1.43	260	48.6	0.07
GARLIC									
raw	100.0	g	149	6.36	33.1	17	401	153	0.5
3 cloves	9.0	g	13.4	0.572	2.98	1.53	36.1	13.8	0.04
GINGER									
raw	100.0	g	80	1.82	17.8	13	415	34	0.75
SPRING ONIONS									
raw	100.0	g	32	1.83	7.34	16	276	37	0.19
1 large	25.0	g	8	0.458	1.84	4	69	9.25	0.04
CHIVES									
raw	100.0	g	30	3.27	4.35	3	296	58	0.73
BASIL									
fresh	100.0	g	23	3.15	2.65	4	295	56	0.64
dried	100.0	g	233	23	47.8	76	2630	274	4.07
OREGANO									
dried	100.0	g	265	9	68.9	25	1260	148	4.28
ROSEMARY									
fresh	100.0	g	131	3.31	20.7	26	668	66	5.86
dried	100.0	g	331	4.88	64.1	50	995	70	15.2
MARJORAM									
dried	100.0	g	271	12.7	60.6	77	1520	306	7.04

SAGE	SERVING QUANTITY	SERVING UNIT	CALORIES (kCal)	PROTEIN (g)	TOTAL CARBOHYDRATES (g)	SODIUM (mg)	POTASSIUM (mg)	PHOSPHORUS (mg)	TOTAL FAT (g)
ground	100.0	g	315	10.6	60.7	11	1070	91	12.8
1 Tbsp	2.0	g	6.3	0.21	1.21	0.22	21.4	1.82	0.25
CINNAMON									
ground	100.0	g	247	3.99	80.6	10	431	64	1.24
1 Tbsp	7.8.0	g	19.3	0.31	6.29	0.78	33.6	4.99	0.09
CUMIN									
seed	100.0	g	375	17.8	44.2	168	1790	499	22.3
1 Tbsp Whole	6.0	g	22.5	1.07	2.65	10.1	107	29.9	1.34
NUTMEG									
ground	100.0	g	525	5.84	49.3	16	350	213	36.3
1 tsp	7.0	g	36.8	0.41	3.45	1.12	24.5	14.9	2.54
CLOVES									
ground	100.0	g	274	5.97	65.5	277	1020	104	13
1tsp	6.5	g	17.8	0.39	4.26	18	66.3	6.76	0.84
PARSLEY									
fresh	100.0	g	36	2.97	6.33	56	554	58	0.79
dried	100.0	g	292	26.6	50.6	452	2680	436	5.48
CORIANDER									
seed	100.0	g	298	12.4	55	35	1270	409	17.8
leaves, raw	100.0	g	23	2.13	3.67	46	521	48	0.52
THYME									
fresh	100.0	g	101	5.56	24.4	9	609	106	1.68
dried	100.0	g	276	9.11	63.9	55	814	201	7.43
LEMON GRASS									
citronella, raw	100.0	g	99	1.82	25.3	6	723	101	0.49

FENNEL	SERVING QUANTITY	SERVING UNIT	CALORIES (kCal)	PROTEIN (g)	TOTAL CARBOHYDRATES (g)	SODIUM (mg)	POTASSIUM (mg)	PHOSPHORUS (mg)	TOTAL FAT (g)
Bulb, raw	100.0	g	31	1.24	7.3	52	414	50	0.2
seed	100.0	g	345	15.8	52.3	88	1690	487	14.9
1 Tbsp	5.8	g	20	0.92	3.03	5.1	98	28	0.86
DILL									
weed, fresh	100.0	g	43	3.46	7.02	61	738	66	1.12
weed, dried	100.0	g	253	20	55.8	208	3310	543	4.36
1 Tbsp	3.1	g	7.8	0.62	1.73	6.45	103	16.8	0.13
ANISE									
seed	100.0	g	337	17.6	50	16	1440	440	15.9
1 Tbsp	6.7	g	22.6	1.18	3.35	1.07	96.5	29.5	1.06
CARDAMOM									
spices	100.0	g	311	10.8	68.5	18	1120	229	6.7
1 Tbsp	5.8	g	18	0.63	3.97	1.04	65	10.3	0.39
CAYENNE									
pepper, red or cayenne	100.0	g	318	12	56.6	30	2010	293	17.3
1 tbsp	5.3	g	16.9	0.64	3	1.59	107	15.5	0.91
CURRY POWDER									
	100.0	g	325	14.3	55.8	52	1170	367	14
1 tbsp	6.3	g	20.5	0.90	3.52	3.28	73.7	23.1	0.88
PAPRIKA									
ground	100.0	g	282	14.1	54	68	2280	314	12.9
1 tbsp	6.8	g	19.2	0.96	3.67	4.62	155	21.4	0.87
CELERY									
celery, raw	100.0	g	14	0.69	2.97	80	260	24	0.17

SAFFRON	SERVING QUANTITY	SERVING UNIT	CALORIES (kCal)	PROTEIN (g)	TOTAL CARBOHYDRATES (g)	SODIUM (mg)	POTASSIUM (mg)	PHOSPHORUS (mg)	TOTAL FAT (g)
	100.0	g	310	11.4	65.4	148	1720	252	5.85
1 tbsp	2.1	g	6.51	0.24	1.37	3.11	36.1	5.29	0.12
PEPPER, BLACK									
ground	100.0	g	251	10.4	64	20	1330	158	3.26
1 tbsp	6.9	g	17.3	0.72	4.42	1.38	91.8	10.9	0.22
PEPPER, WHITE									
ground	100.0	g	296	10.4	68.6	5	73	176	2.12
1 tbsp	7.1	g	21	0.74	4.87	0.35	5.18	12.5	0.15
TARRAGON									
dried	100.0	g	295	22.8	50.2	62	3020	313	7.24
1 Tbsp, leaves	1.8	g	5.31	0.41	0.90	1.12	54.4	5.63	0.13
1 Tbsp, ground	4.8	g	14.2	1.09	2.41	2.98	145	15	0.34
HORSERADISH									
	100.0	g	48	1.18	11.3	420	246	31	0.69
1 tbsp	15.0	g	7.2	0.18	1.7	63	36.9	4.65	0.10

Your Thoughts Matter!

Thank you for taking the time to read this far into *GERD Diet Essentials*. I truly hope the information and recipes have been helpful on your journey to managing GERD.

If you're finding value in this book, I would be incredibly grateful if you could take a few moments to share your thoughts with other readers on Amazon. Your honest review helps others discover this resource and can make a real difference.

You can easily leave a review here:

https://go.binnovatedigital.com/GERDFoodlist

(Scan the QR code below to go directly to the review page):

Thank you so much for your support!

Love,

-Catherine

Chapter 5: Nourishing Your Gut: Delicious and Gentle Recipes for GERD Relief

Welcome to the heart of your journey towards managing GERD: the kitchen! As a fellow traveler on this path, and your dedicated gastro nurse, I understand firsthand the delicate dance between enjoying delicious food and finding relief from those unwelcome reflux symptoms. For too long, many of my patients have felt restricted and overwhelmed by what they *can't* eat. This chapter is here to flip that script.

Think of this not as a list of limitations, but as an invitation to explore a vibrant world of flavors and textures that can be both satisfying and kind to your digestive system. The recipes you'll find in this chapter are crafted with your comfort in mind. They prioritize ingredients and cooking methods that are generally well-tolerated by those with GERD, focusing on lower acidity, moderate healthy fats, and avoiding common triggers that can send that familiar burn creeping up.

Remember, managing GERD is a multifaceted approach, and diet plays a crucial role. While these recipes offer a solid foundation, listening to your own body and understanding your personal triggers remains paramount. Consider this chapter your starting point – a collection of delicious and gentle meals and snacks that can empower you to take control of your dietary choices and rediscover the joy of eating without the fear of discomfort.

Each recipe includes not only a simple step-by-step guide but also insights into why it's considered GERD-friendly and any specific precautions you might want to consider. We'll delve into the nutritional benefits, helping you understand how these choices contribute to your overall well-being.

So, let's put on our aprons and embark on this culinary adventure together. It's time to nourish your gut, soothe your esophagus, and rediscover the pleasure of a delicious, symptom-friendly meal. You deserve to enjoy food without the fight, and these recipes are designed to help you do just that. Happy cooking!

Breakfast Ideas

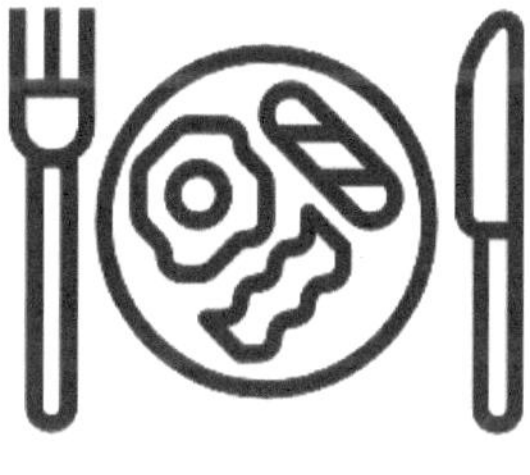

Oatmeal with Bananas and Almonds

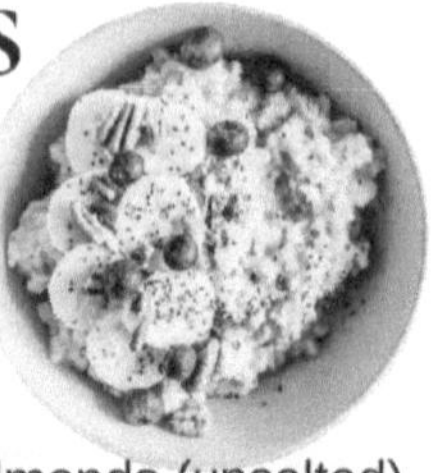

Ingredients

- 1 cup rolled oats (gluten-free if needed)
- 2 cups water or unsweetened almond milk (for cooking oats)
- 1 medium banana (sliced)
- 1/4 cup sliced almonds (unsalted)
- 1 tablespoon honey or maple syrup (optional, adjust based on sweetness preference)
- 1/2 teaspoon ground cinnamon (optional)
- Pinch of salt (optional)

Directions

1. Cook Oats: In a saucepan, bring 2 cups of water or almond milk to a boil. Stir in the rolled oats, reduce the heat to low, and simmer for about 5-7 minutes, stirring occasionally until the oats are tender and the liquid is absorbed.
2. Prepare Bananas: While the oatmeal is cooking, slice the banana.
3. Mix in Ingredients: Once the oatmeal is cooked, remove it from heat. Stir in the sliced banana, sliced almonds, honey (or maple syrup, if using), cinnamon (if using), and a pinch of salt (if desired).
4. Serve: Divide the oatmeal into bowls and enjoy warm.

1 serving: Approximately 1 cup of oatmeal.

Nutritional Information per Serving

- Calories: 300 kcal (approximately; varies based on almond milk and sweetener)
- Carbohydrates: 50 g
- Fat: 10 g (varies with almonds and almond milk)
- Protein: 8 g
- Potassium: 400 mg (may vary based on banana and almond milk)
- Phosphorus: 120 mg
- Sodium: 5 mg (depending on added salt)

Why is this good for you?

- *Gentle on the Stomach: Oatmeal is a soothing, high-fiber food that can help absorb stomach acid and reduce symptoms of GERD. It is also low in fat, which is beneficial for managing GERD symptoms.*
- *Nutrient-Rich: Bananas are low in acidity and provide potassium, which can help maintain electrolyte balance. Almonds add healthy fats and protein, making the meal more satisfying.*
- *Customizable: This recipe can be easily adjusted with different toppings or sweeteners based on individual preferences and dietary restrictions, allowing for a variety of flavors without triggering GERD symptoms.*

SPECIAL PRECAUTIONS!

Monitor portion sizes of bananas and almonds to manage potassium intake, especially for individuals who need to restrict potassium.

Adjust sweetness based on individual dietary restrictions, and consult with a healthcare provider or dietitian for personalized dietary advice.

Smoothie Bowl with Spinach and Berries

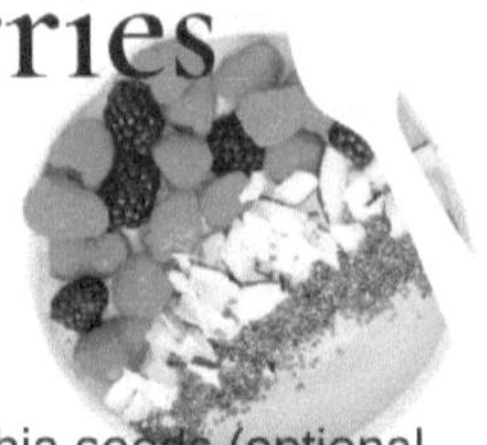

Ingredients

- 1 cup fresh spinach (washed)
- 1 cup mixed berries (fresh or frozen; e.g., strawberries, blueberries, raspberries)
- 1 medium banana (preferably frozen for creaminess)
- 1 cup unsweetened almond milk (or any low-sodium milk alternative)
- 1 tablespoon chia seeds (optional, for added fiber and omega-3)
- 1 tablespoon honey or maple syrup (optional, adjust based on sweetness preference)

Toppings (optional):
- 1/4 cup granola (low-sugar)
- Sliced fresh fruit (e.g., banana, kiwi)
- Nuts or seeds (e.g., sliced almonds, pumpkin seeds)

Directions

1. Blend Ingredients: In a blender, combine the fresh spinach, mixed berries, banana, and unsweetened almond milk. If using, add chia seeds and honey or maple syrup for sweetness.
2. Blend Until Smooth: Blend on high speed until the mixture is smooth and creamy. If the smoothie is too thick, add a little more almond milk until you reach your desired consistency.
3. Serve: Pour the smoothie into a bowl. Top with your choice of granola, sliced fresh fruit, and nuts or seeds.
4. Enjoy: Serve immediately as a nutritious breakfast or snack.

1 serving: Approximately 1 cup of smoothie bowl

Nutritional Information per Serving

- Calories: 250 kcal (approximately; varies based on toppings and sweetener)
- Carbohydrates: 40 g
- Fat: 8 g (varies with almond milk and toppings)
- Protein: 6 g
- Potassium: 450 mg (may vary based on fruits and spinach)
- Phosphorus: 80 mg
- Sodium: 50 mg (depending on almond milk and toppings)

Why is this good for you?

- *Gentle on the Stomach: The ingredients in this smoothie bowl are low in acidity, making it a soothing option for those with GERD. Spinach and berries are both nutrient-dense and easy to digest.*
- *Nutrient-Rich: Spinach provides vitamins A, C, and K, while berries are rich in antioxidants. The combination supports overall health without triggering GERD symptoms.*
- *Customizable: This recipe can be easily adjusted with different fruits and toppings based on individual preferences and dietary restrictions, allowing for a variety of flavors without excessive acidity.*

SPECIAL PRECAUTIONS!

Monitor portion sizes of bananas and berries to manage potassium intake, especially for individuals who need to restrict potassium.

Adjust sweetness based on individual dietary restrictions and consult with a healthcare provider or dietitian for personalized dietary advice.

Lunch Options

GERD-Friendly Quinoa Salad with Cucumbers and Chickpeas

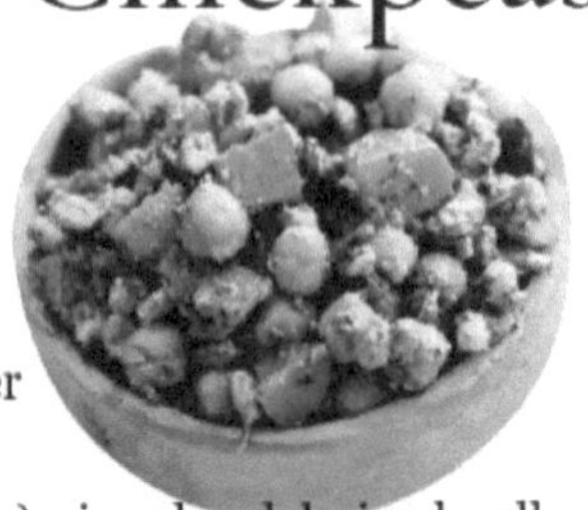

Ingredients

- For the Salad:
- 1 cup dry quinoa, rinsed thoroughly under cold water
- 2 cups water or low-sodium vegetable broth[2]
- 1 can (15-ounce / ~425g) chickpeas (garbanzo beans), rinsed and drained well
- 1 large cucumber, peeled (optional), seeded, and diced (about 1.5 - 2 cups)
- 1 medium red bell pepper, deseeded and finely diced (optional, adds color and nutrients)
- 1/2 cup chopped fresh parsley (or dill, or a mix)
- For the Dressing:
- 2 tablespoons extra virgin olive oil
- 1 tablespoon fresh lemon juice (Optional - start with less or omit if sensitive to acidity)
- 1/4 teaspoon salt (or to taste – use sparingly)
- Pinch of black pepper (omit if sensitive)

Directions

1. Cook the Quinoa: In a medium saucepan, combine the rinsed quinoa and water/broth. Bring to a boil, then reduce heat to low, cover, and simmer for 15-20 minutes, or until all liquid is absorbed and the quinoa is cooked (it should look slightly translucent with the outer germ ring visible). Fluff with a fork and let it cool completely. You can spread it on a baking sheet to speed up cooling.
2. Prepare Vegetables & Chickpeas: While the quinoa cooks/cools, prepare the cucumber, bell pepper (if using), and parsley. Ensure the chickpeas are well-rinsed to remove excess sodium.
3. Make the Dressing: In a small bowl or jar, whisk together the olive oil, lemon juice (if using - start with 1-2 teaspoons and taste), salt, and pepper (if using).
4. Combine: In a large bowl, combine the cooled quinoa, rinsed chickpeas, diced cucumber, diced red bell pepper (if using), and chopped parsley.
5. Dress the Salad: Pour the dressing over the salad ingredients. Gently toss everything together until well combined.
6. Chill (Optional): For best flavor, you can chill the salad in the refrigerator for about 15-30 minutes before serving, but it can also be eaten immediately.

Servings: Approximately 4 servings

Nutritional Information per Serving

- Calories: ~320-350 kcal
- Carbohydrates: ~45-50 g
- Protein: ~11-13 g
- Fat: ~11-13 g (primarily unsaturated fat from olive oil and quinoa)
- Potassium: ~450-550 mg
- Sodium: ~200-250 mg (will vary based on added salt and canned chickpeas rinsing effectiveness)
- Phosphorus: ~300-350 mg

Why is this good for you?

- *Low Fat: The recipe uses minimal added fat (olive oil), and avoids high-fat ingredients like creamy dressings, cheese, or fatty meats, which can slow digestion and relax the LES.*
- *High Fiber: Quinoa, chickpeas, cucumbers, and bell peppers provide dietary fiber, which aids digestion and can promote feelings of fullness, potentially helping prevent overeating (a GERD trigger).*
- *Low Acidity: Uses minimal or optional lemon juice. It avoids highly acidic ingredients like tomatoes or vinegar-heavy dressings. Cucumber is a high-water, low-acid vegetable.*
- *Excludes Common Irritants: Free from common GERD triggers like onions, garlic, excessive spice, and mint.*

SPECIAL PRECAUTIONS!

- Chickpea Rinsing: Rinse canned chickpeas very well under running water to significantly reduce their sodium content.
- Lemon Juice Sensitivity: Lemon juice is acidic. Start with a very small amount (1 tsp) or omit it completely if you are sensitive to acidic foods. You can rely on the olive oil and fresh herbs for flavour.

Grilled Chicken & Spinach Wrap

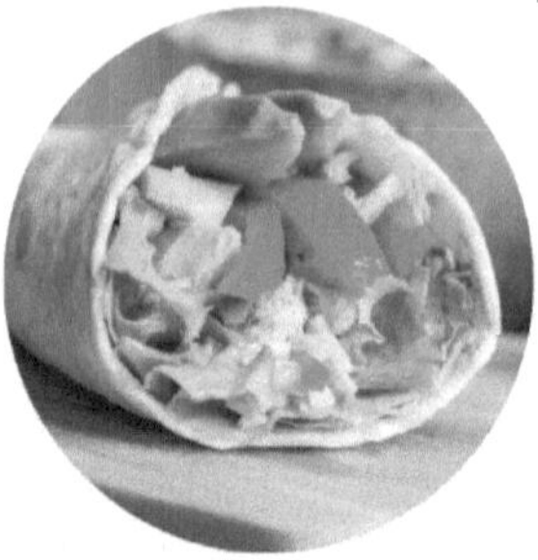

Ingredients

For the Chicken:

- 6 oz (about 170g) boneless, skinless chicken breast
- 1 teaspoon olive oil
- Pinch of salt
- Pinch of black pepper (omit if sensitive)
- 1/4 teaspoon dried oregano or thyme (optional, avoid garlic/onion powder)

For the Wrap & Filling:

- 2 medium (8-inch) whole wheat tortillas (or soft white flour tortillas if whole wheat causes issues for you)
- 2 cups fresh baby spinach
- 1/2 cup shredded carrots
- 1/2 cup thinly sliced cucumber
- 1/4 cup thinly sliced red bell pepper (optional)

For the Binder (Choose ONE or use a mix sparingly):

- 1/4 ripe avocado, mashed well (use sparingly due to fat content)
- OR 1/4 cup plain, low-fat Greek yogurt (ensure no high-acid additives)

Directions

1. Prepare the Chicken: Pat the chicken breast dry. Rub it with olive oil, salt, pepper (if using), and dried herbs (if using).
2. Grill the Chicken: Cook the chicken breast on a preheated grill (outdoor or indoor grill pan) over medium heat for about 5-7 minutes per side, or until cooked through (internal temperature reaches 165°F / 74°C). Let the chicken rest for 5 minutes, then slice or shred it.
3. Warm Tortillas (Optional): Briefly warm the tortillas in a dry skillet, microwave, or oven to make them more pliable.
4. Assemble the Wraps:Lay a tortilla flat.
    a. Spread your chosen binder (mashed avocado OR Greek yogurt) thinly over the center of the tortilla, leaving a border around the edges.
    b. Layer the fresh spinach over the binder.
    c. Top with the cooked chicken slices/shreds.
    d. Add the shredded carrots, sliced cucumber, and red bell pepper (if using).
5. Wrap it Up: Fold in the sides of the tortilla first, then tightly roll it up from the bottom. Slice in half if desired.
6. Serve: Serve immediately.

Servings: 2 wraps

Nutritional Information per Serving

- Calories: ~350-380 kcal
- Carbohydrates: ~30-35 g
- Protein: ~30-33 g
- Fat: ~10-12 g (using 1/8 avocado per wrap; will be lower if using Greek yogurt)
- Potassium: ~550-650 mg
- Sodium: ~350-450 mg (highly dependent on tortilla brand and added salt)
- Phosphorus: ~300-350 mg

Why is this good for you?

- *Lean Protein: Grilled chicken breast is low in fat, supporting muscle health without typically triggering reflux associated with fatty meats.*
- *Low Fat Binder Options: Offers mashed avocado (healthy fats, use sparingly) or low-fat Greek yogurt, avoiding high-fat mayonnaise or creamy dressings.*
- *Gentle Vegetables: Spinach, carrots, and cucumbers are generally well-tolerated, low-acid vegetables.*
- *No Common Irritants: Free from garlic, onions, spicy seasonings, tomatoes, and excessive acidity.*
- *Fiber: Whole wheat tortillas (if used) and vegetables contribute fiber, aiding digestion.*

SPECIAL PRECAUTIONS!

- Individual Triggers: Monitor your tolerance. Some might find even bell peppers or whole wheat tortillas problematic.
- Avocado Moderation: Avocado is a source of healthy fat, but fat can still be a trigger for some. Use it sparingly (e.g., 1/8th of a medium avocado per wrap). If fat is a major trigger, low-fat Greek yogurt is likely a safer binder choice.
- Chicken Preparation: Ensure chicken is cooked through but not overly charred, as heavily charred bits can sometimes be irritating.

Dinner Recipes

Baked Salmon with Asparagus

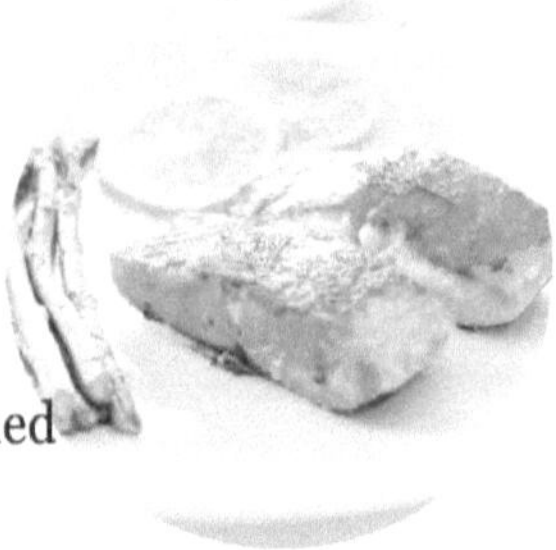

Ingredients

- 2 (4-6 ounce) salmon fillets, skin on or off
- 1 bunch (about 1 pound) asparagus spears, trimmed
- 1 tablespoon olive oil (a healthy fat)
- 1 tablespoon fresh lemon juice (use sparingly, see precautions)
- 1 teaspoon dried dill (a mild, GERD-friendly herb)
- ½ teaspoon garlic powder (less likely to cause issues than fresh garlic for some)
- Salt to taste (use moderately)
- Fresh parsley, chopped (for garnish, optional)

Directions

1. Preheat the oven: Preheat your oven to 400°F (200°C).
2. Prepare the asparagus: Toss the trimmed asparagus spears in a bowl with ½ tablespoon of olive oil and a pinch of salt. Spread them in a single layer on a baking sheet.
3. Prepare the salmon: Pat the salmon fillets dry with paper towels. Place them on the same baking sheet as the asparagus, ensuring they are not overcrowded.
4. Season the salmon: Drizzle the salmon fillets with the remaining ½ tablespoon of olive oil and the lemon juice. Sprinkle with dried dill, garlic powder, and salt.
5. Bake: Bake for 12-15 minutes, or until the salmon is cooked through and flakes easily with a fork, and the asparagus is tender-crisp. Cooking time will vary depending on the thickness of the salmon and asparagus.
6. Serve: Carefully remove the baking sheet from the oven. Garnish with fresh parsley, if desired, and serve immediately.

Servings: 2

Nutritional Information per Serving

- Calories: 250-350 (depending on salmon fat content and portion size)
- Carbohydrates: 5-7 grams
- Protein: 30-40 grams
- Fat: 12-20 grams (mostly healthy unsaturated fats from salmon and olive oil)
- Potassium: 500-700 mg (estimated, primarily from salmon and asparagus)
- Sodium: Varies depending on added salt
- Phosphorus: 300-450 mg (estimated, primarily from salmon and asparagus)

Why is this good for you?

- *Healthy Fats: Olive oil is a source of healthy monounsaturated fats, which are less likely to trigger GERD symptoms compared to saturated and trans fats found in fried foods or fatty meats.*
- *Low Acidity: While lemon juice is used, the amount is minimal. For some individuals highly sensitive to acidic foods, it can be omitted or substituted with a very mild alternative like a small amount of diluted apple cider vinegar (use with caution and in very small quantities).*
- *Moderate Fat Content: The overall fat content is moderate, which helps with digestion and reduces the likelihood of delayed stomach emptying.*

SPECIAL PRECAUTIONS!

- Lemon Juice: While a small amount of lemon juice is used for flavor, some individuals with severe GERD may be sensitive to citrus. If you find lemon to be a trigger, omit it entirely or use a very small amount and monitor your symptoms. You could try a tiny splash of a very mild vinegar (like rice vinegar) or simply rely on the herbs for flavor.
- Garlic: While garlic powder is often better tolerated than fresh garlic, some individuals may still find it irritating. If garlic is a trigger for you, omit it.

Vegetable Stir-Fry with Tofu

Ingredients

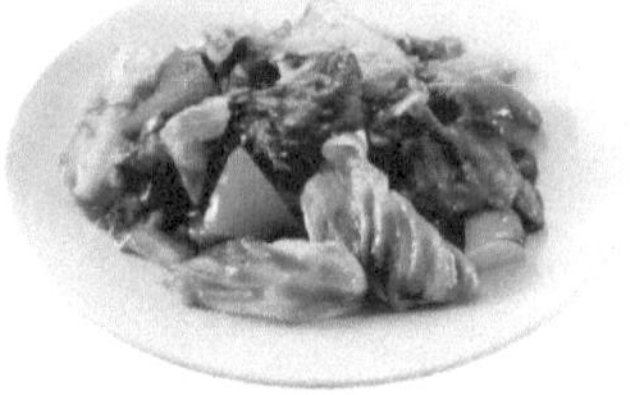

- 1 block (14-16 ounces) extra-firm tofu, pressed to remove excess water
- 1 tablespoon olive oil (a healthier fat)
- Assorted GERD-friendly vegetables, about 4-6 cups total, chopped into bite-sized pieces (suggestions below)
- For the Sauce:2 tablespoons low-sodium soy sauce or tamari (for gluten-free)
- 1 tablespoon rice vinegar (use cautiously, see precautions)
- 1 teaspoon maple syrup or a very small amount of honey (optional, for mild sweetness)
- ½ teaspoon cornstarch or arrowroot powder (to thicken)
- ½ teaspoon grated fresh ginger (use sparingly, see precautions)
- 1 small clove garlic, minced (use sparingly, see precautions)
- ½ teaspoon sesame oil (optional, for flavor)
- Pinch of mild dried herbs like thyme or oregano (optional, instead of pepper)
- Cooked white rice or rice noodles (less acidic than some other grains), for serving (optional)
- Sesame seeds or finely chopped green onion tops (green parts only), for garnish (optional)

GERD-Friendly Vegetable Suggestions:

- Broccoli florets (well-cooked)
- Carrots, sliced or julienned
- Bell peppers (yellow or orange are often better tolerated than red), sliced
- Snap peas or snow peas
- Mushrooms, sliced
- Green beans, trimmed
- Zucchini or yellow squash, sliced
- Asparagus, chopped
- Spinach or other mild leafy greens (added towards the end)

Servings: 2 -4

Directions

1. Prepare the Tofu: Cut the pressed tofu into cubes or triangles. You can toss it with ½ teaspoon of cornstarch for a slightly crispier texture if desired.
2. Make the Sauce: In a small bowl, whisk together the low-sodium soy sauce (or tamari), rice vinegar, maple syrup (or honey, if using), cornstarch (or arrowroot powder), ginger, garlic, sesame oil (if using), and dried herbs (if using). Set aside.

Directions cont...

3. Cook the Tofu: Heat the olive oil in a large skillet, wok, or non-stick pan over medium heat (avoiding high heat that can burn and create potential irritants). Add the tofu and cook gently, stirring occasionally, until lightly golden on all sides (about 5-7 minutes). Remove the tofu from the pan and set aside.
4. Stir-fry the Vegetables: Add the harder vegetables (like carrots and broccoli) to the pan first and stir-fry for 3-4 minutes until slightly tender-crisp. Then, add the softer vegetables (like bell peppers, mushrooms, and green beans) and continue to stir-fry for another 3-5 minutes until all the vegetables are tender but not mushy. Add spinach or other leafy greens in the last minute until just wilted. Add a tablespoon of water or vegetable broth if the pan gets too dry.
5. Combine and Thicken: Return the cooked tofu to the pan with the vegetables. Stir the sauce again and pour it over the tofu and vegetables. Cook, stirring gently, for 1-2 minutes until the sauce thickens slightly and coats everything evenly.
6. Serve: Serve the GERD-friendly vegetable stir-fry with tofu immediately over cooked white rice or rice noodles, if desired. Garnish with sesame seeds or finely chopped green onion tops.

Nutritional Information per Serving

(based on 4 servings, using a variety of suggested vegetables and a basic sauce, without rice/noodles):

- Calories: 180-280 (estimation will vary greatly based on the amount and type of vegetables and oil used)
- Carbohydrates: 12-20 grams
- Protein: 9-14 grams
- Fat: 9-14 grams (mostly healthy unsaturated fats from olive and sesame oil, and tofu)
- Potassium: Varies widely depending on vegetables used (carrots, broccoli, spinach are good sources)
- Sodium: Varies depending on the amount of low-sodium soy sauce used
- Phosphorus: Varies depending on tofu and vegetables used

Snack Ideas

GERD-Friendly Hummus with Carrot Sticks

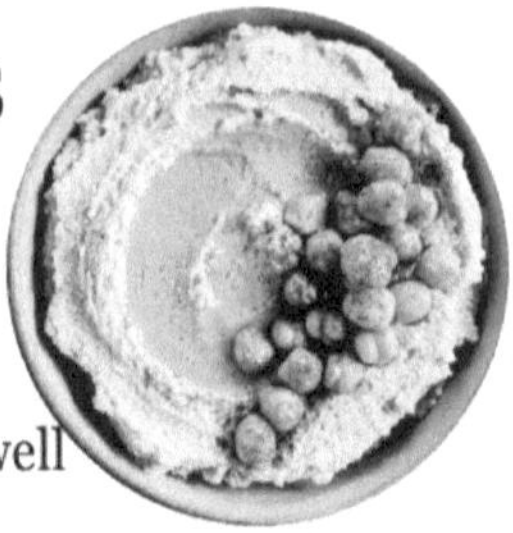

Ingredients

For the Hummus:

- 1 (15-ounce) can chickpeas, rinsed and drained well
- ¼ cup tahini (sesame seed paste)
- 2-3 tablespoons cold water (adjust to desired consistency)
- 1-2 tablespoons olive oil (a healthy fat)
- 1 tablespoon fresh lemon juice (use sparingly, see precautions)
- ½ small clove garlic, minced (use very sparingly or omit, see precautions)
- ¼ teaspoon ground cumin (a milder spice)
- Pinch of salt (use moderately)

Servings: 6-8

For Serving: 1 pound carrots, peeled and cut into sticks

Directions

1. Prepare the Chickpeas: Ensure the chickpeas are thoroughly rinsed and drained. This can help with digestibility.
2. Combine Ingredients: In a food processor, combine the rinsed and drained chickpeas and tahini. Process for about 1-2 minutes, scraping down the sides occasionally, until the mixture is smooth and creamy.
3. Add Liquids: With the food processor running, slowly drizzle in the cold water and olive oil until the hummus reaches your desired smooth and creamy consistency. Start with less water and add more as needed.
4. Add Flavorings: Add the lemon juice, minced garlic (if using), cumin, and salt. Process for another 30 seconds until everything is well combined. Taste and adjust seasoning if needed, being mindful of potential GERD triggers. You might prefer less garlic or lemon juice than in traditional hummus.
5. Chill: Transfer the hummus to a serving bowl, cover, and chill in the refrigerator for at least 30 minutes to allow the flavors to meld. Chilling can also make it slightly thicker.
6. Prepare Carrot Sticks: While the hummus is chilling, peel the carrots and cut them into sticks.
7. Serve: Serve the chilled GERD-friendly hummus with the prepared carrot sticks for dipping

Nutritional Information per Serving

- Calories: 120-150
- Carbohydrates: 14-18 grams
- Protein: 4-6 grams
- Fat: 7-9 grams (mostly healthy unsaturated fats)
- Potassium: 150-250 mg (estimated, primarily from chickpeas and carrots)
- Sodium: Varies depending on added salt and sodium content of canned chickpeas (rinsing helps reduce sodium)
- Phosphorus: 80-120 mg (estimated, primarily from chickpeas)

Why is this good for you?

- *Lean Protein and Fiber: Chickpeas provide a good source of plant-based protein and fiber, which can promote satiety and aid digestion without the high fat content found in some other dips.*
- *Healthy Fats: Olive oil and tahini contain healthy unsaturated fats, which are generally better tolerated than saturated and trans fats. The amount of olive oil is moderate.*
- *Lower Acidity: This recipe uses a smaller amount of lemon juice compared to traditional hummus recipes. For those highly sensitive to acidic foods, the lemon juice can be further reduced or even omitted, though it does contribute to the flavor.*

SPECIAL PRECAUTIONS!

- Lemon Juice: Even a small amount of lemon juice can be problematic for some individuals with GERD. If you find lemon to be a trigger, start with a very small amount (e.g., ½ teaspoon) and see how you tolerate it, or omit it entirely. You might try a tiny splash of a very mild vinegar (like rice vinegar) or simply rely on the other flavors.
- Garlic: Garlic is a common GERD trigger. This recipe recommends using a very small amount or omitting it. Pay attention to your body's reaction.
- Tahini: While generally well-tolerated, tahini is relatively high in fat. The amount in this recipe is moderate, but be mindful of your overall fat intake.

Greek Yogurt with Honey and Nuts

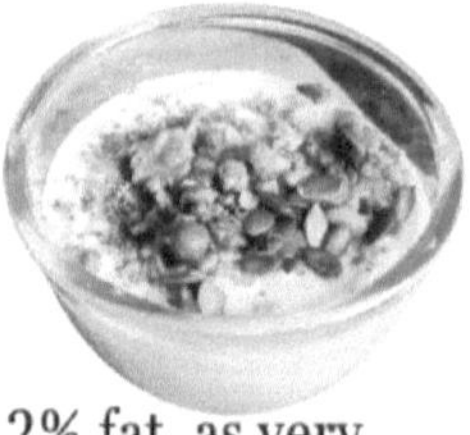

Ingredients

- 1 cup plain Greek yogurt (preferably full-fat or 2% fat, as very low-fat options might empty from the stomach more quickly for some individuals)
- 1 teaspoon honey (use sparingly, see precautions)
- 1-2 tablespoons chopped nuts (such as almonds, walnuts, or pecans - avoid high-fat nuts like macadamia in large quantities if fat is a trigger)

Serving: 1

Directions

1. Spoon Yogurt: Spoon the Greek yogurt into a bowl.
2. Drizzle Honey: Drizzle the honey evenly over the yogurt.
3. Sprinkle Nuts: Sprinkle the chopped nuts over the yogurt and honey.
4. Serve: Enjoy immediately.

Nutritional Information per Serving

- Calories: 250-300
- Carbohydrates: 15-20 grams (from yogurt, honey, and nuts)
- Protein: 20-25 grams (primarily from Greek yogurt and nuts)
- Fat: 12-18 grams (mostly healthy fats from yogurt and nuts)
- Potassium: 300-400 mg (estimated, primarily from Greek yogurt and almonds)
- Sodium: 80-100 mg (estimated, varies based on the yogurt brand)
- Phosphorus: 200-250 mg (estimated, primarily from Greek yogurt and almonds)

Why is this good for you?

- *High Protein: Greek yogurt is a good source of protein, which can promote feelings of fullness and may aid in stomach emptying at a steady rate.*
- *Lower Acidity (compared to regular yogurt): Greek yogurt undergoes a straining process that removes whey, resulting in a thicker texture and generally lower lactose and slightly lower acidity compared to regular yogurt.*
- *Healthy Fats (in moderation): The healthy fats from full-fat or 2% fat Greek yogurt and nuts can contribute to satiety without being overly heavy. Very low-fat options might empty from the stomach too quickly for some, potentially increasing reflux.*
- *Mild Sweetness: Honey provides a natural and generally well-tolerated sweetener when used in moderation.*
- *Good Source of Calcium and Probiotics: Greek yogurt is a good source of calcium and often contains probiotics, which may contribute to gut health (though the direct impact on GERD is still being researched).*

SPECIAL PRECAUTIONS!

- Honey: While generally better tolerated than processed sugars for some, honey is still a simple sugar and can contribute to reflux in some individuals if consumed in large amounts. Use it sparingly and monitor your symptoms.
- Nuts: Nuts are generally healthy but can be high in fat. While healthy fats are usually better than unhealthy fats, consuming large amounts of any fat can delay stomach emptying and potentially worsen reflux for some. Stick to the recommended serving size and choose nuts that are well-tolerated. Avoid nuts that are heavily processed or seasoned with strong spices.
- Fat Content: While full-fat or 2% Greek yogurt might be better for some regarding stomach emptying, individuals who are sensitive to fat as a GERD trigger might need to opt for a lower-fat option and monitor their symptoms.
- Timing of Consumption: Be mindful of when you consume this snack. Avoid eating it right before lying down, as this can increase the risk of reflux.

Chapter 6: Meal Planning for Success: Your Blueprint for Delicious, Heartburn-Free Eating

You've learned about GERD, understood the basics of a GERD-friendly diet, and explored lists of foods to enjoy and those to approach with caution. Now, let's put that knowledge into action! This chapter will guide you through the practical steps of meal planning, equipping you with strategies to create a weekly roadmap of delicious and symptom-friendly meals. With a little planning, you can take control of your diet, reduce the stress of last-minute food decisions, and set yourself up for long-term success in managing your GERD.

How to Create a Weekly Meal Plan: Your Step-by-Step Guide

Creating a weekly meal plan might seem daunting at first, but it's a powerful tool for staying on track with your GERD diet and ensuring you always have nourishing, safe options available. Here's a simple step-by-step approach:

1. Assess Your Week: Take a look at your schedule for the upcoming week. Consider how many meals you'll need to plan for, any busy evenings where quick meals are essential, and any social events or dining out you might have.

2. Brainstorm GERD-Friendly Meals: Think about the GERD-friendly foods you enjoy and the types of meals you typically eat (breakfast, lunch, dinner, snacks). Refer back to the "Foods to Embrace" list in Chapter 3 and any recipes you've found in this book or elsewhere. Jot down a variety of meal ideas.

3. Check Your Pantry and Fridge: Before creating your plan, take inventory of what you already have on hand. This will help you avoid buying unnecessary ingredients and inspire meal ideas based on what you need to use up.

4. Select Your Meals for Each Day: Based on your schedule and the ingredients you have or need, start assigning meals to specific days. Aim for a balance of different types of meals throughout the week. Consider themes (e.g., "Meatless Monday," "Fish Friday") if that helps you organize.

5. Plan Your Main Courses First: Dinner is often the most involved meal, so start by planning your main courses for the week. Once those are set, you can build your lunches and breakfasts around them, potentially using leftovers.

6. Incorporate Sides and Snacks: Don't forget to plan your side dishes to complement your main meals. Also, think about healthy, GERD-friendly snacks you can have on

hand for between meals to prevent overeating at mealtimes.

7. Create Your Grocery List: Once your meal plan is complete, create a detailed grocery list of all the ingredients you'll need. Organize your list by grocery store sections (e.g., produce, dairy, meats) to make shopping more efficient.

8. Be Flexible: Life happens! Don't be afraid to swap meals around if your schedule changes or if you're not in the mood for something you planned. The goal is to have a framework, not a rigid set of rules.

9. Review and Adjust: At the end of the week, take a moment to review how well your meal plan worked. Did you enjoy the meals? Were they GERD-friendly? Make notes of what worked well and what you might want to change for the following week.

Tips for Meal Prepping GERD-Friendly Meals: Your Time-Saving Secret Weapon

Meal prepping – preparing meals or components of meals in advance – can be a game-changer for managing your GERD diet, especially on busy days. Here are some tips to make meal prepping work for you:

- Dedicate Time for Prep: Choose a day or two each week (e.g., Sunday and Wednesday) to dedicate a few hours to meal prepping.
- Focus on Components: You don't have to prepare entire meals. Sometimes prepping individual components like

cooked grains, roasted vegetables, or grilled chicken can save significant time during the week.

- Double Recipes: When you're cooking a GERD-friendly meal, consider making a double batch. You can enjoy the leftovers for lunch the next day or freeze portions for future quick meals.
- Portion Control: Meal prepping is a great way to practice portion control, which is crucial for managing GERD symptoms. Portion out your meals into individual containers.
- Invest in Good Containers: Having a variety of airtight containers in different sizes will make storing and transporting your prepped meals much easier.
- Wash and Chop Produce: Spend some time washing, chopping, and storing your fruits and vegetables. This makes it quick to add them to salads, stir-fries, or snacks during the week.
- Prepare Breakfast in Advance: Overnight oats, hard-boiled eggs, or pre-portioned smoothie ingredients can make busy mornings much smoother.
- Label Everything: Clearly label your containers with the contents and the date they were prepared to ensure freshness and avoid food waste.
- Store Properly: Be sure to store your prepped meals at the correct temperature in the refrigerator or freezer to maintain food safety.

Sample One-Week GERD Meal Plan: A Starting Point for Inspiration

This is just a sample meal plan to give you an idea of how to structure your week. Remember to adjust it based on your individual preferences, dietary needs, and tolerance levels.

Monday

- Breakfast:
  Oatmeal (½ cup dry) with sliced banana (1 medium) and a drizzle of honey (1 tsp).
- Lunch:
  Leftover Baked Chicken Breast (4 oz) with Roasted Carrots (1 cup) and Green Beans (1 cup).
- Dinner:
  Baked Salmon (4 oz) with Quinoa (½ cup cooked) and Steamed Broccoli (1 cup).
- Snacks:
  Rice cakes (2) with avocado (¼ medium), a small pear (1).
- Estimated Daily Macros:
  - Calories: ~1500-1700 kcal
  - Carbohydrates: ~180-220 g
  - Proteins: ~90-110 g
  - Fats: ~40-60 g
  - Sodium: ~300-500 mg
  - Potassium: ~2500-3000 mg
  - Phosphorus: ~800-1000 mg

Tuesday

- Breakfast:
  Smoothie made with spinach (1 cup), banana (1 medium), almond milk (1 cup unsweetened), and plain low-fat yogurt (½ cup).
- Lunch:
  Turkey Breast (4 oz) and Lettuce Wraps (3-4 leaves) with sliced cucumber (½ cup).
- Dinner:
  Lean Ground Turkey Stir-fry (4 oz) with brown rice (½ cup cooked) and mixed non-acidic vegetables (bell peppers ½ cup, zucchini ½ cup).
- Snacks:
  A handful of almonds (¼ cup), a small melon wedge (1 cup).
- Estimated Daily Macros:
  - Calories: ~1400-1600 kcal
  - Carbohydrates: ~150-190 g
  - Proteins: ~100-120 g
  - Fats: ~40-55 g
  - Sodium: ~400-600 mg
  - Potassium: ~2800-3300 mg
  - Phosphorus: ~900-1100 mg

Wednesday

- Breakfast:
  Scrambled egg whites (3) with a side of whole-wheat toast (1 slice).
- Lunch:
  Leftover Lean Ground Turkey Stir-fry (same as Tuesday dinner).
- Dinner:
  Baked Chicken Breast (4 oz) and Potato (1 medium) Foil Packets with herbs (no onions or garlic if they are triggers). Steamed green beans (½ cup).
- Snacks:
  Plain low-fat yogurt (½ cup), a few strawberries (½ cup).
- Estimated Daily Macros:
  - Calories: ~1300-1500 kcal
  - Carbohydrates: ~140-170 g
  - Proteins: ~90-110 g
  - Fats: ~30-45 g
  - Sodium: ~350-550 mg
  - Potassium: ~2600-3100 mg
  - Phosphorus: ~850-1050 mg

Thursday

- Breakfast:
  Whole-wheat toast (1 slice) with mashed avocado (¼ medium).
- Lunch:
  Salad with grilled chicken breast (4 oz), mixed greens (2 cups), cucumber (½ cup), and a light vinaigrette dressing (2 tbsp).
- Dinner:
  Lentil Soup (1.5 cups) with a side of whole-grain bread (1 slice).
- Snacks:
  A small banana (1), a few walnuts (¼ cup).
- Estimated Daily Macros:
  - Calories: ~1400-1600 kcal
  - Carbohydrates: ~160-200 g
  - Proteins: ~80-100 g
  - Fats: ~50-70 g
  - Sodium: ~500-700 mg
  - Potassium: ~2900-3400 mg
  - Phosphorus: ~750-950 mg

Friday

- Breakfast:
  Overnight oats (½ cup dry) with berries (½ cup).
- Lunch:
  Leftover Lentil Soup (same as Thursday dinner).
- Dinner:
  Baked Cod (4 oz) with roasted sweet potatoes (1 medium) and steamed asparagus (1 cup).
- Snacks:
  Rice cakes (2) with a thin layer of almond butter (1 tbsp), a small apple (1).
- Estimated Daily Macros:
  - Calories: ~1500-1700 kcal
  - Carbohydrates: ~190-230 g
  - Proteins: ~90-110 g
  - Fats: ~40-60 g
  - Sodium: ~400-600 mg
  - Potassium: ~3000-3500 mg
  - Phosphorus: ~950-1150 mg

Saturday

- Breakfast:
  Scrambled eggs (2) with diced bell peppers (½ cup, if tolerated).
- Lunch:
  Tuna salad (4 oz tuna, 2 tbsp low-fat mayonnaise) on lettuce cups (3-4 leaves).
- Dinner:
  Homemade Chicken (4 oz) and Vegetable Skewers (1 cup mixed GERD-friendly vegetables) grilled or baked.
- Snacks:
  A small pear (1), a handful of cashews (¼ cup).
- Estimated Daily Macros:
  - Calories: ~1400-1600 kcal
  - Carbohydrates: ~130-170 g
  - Proteins: ~100-120 g
  - Fats: ~50-70 g
  - Sodium: ~450-650 mg
  - Potassium: ~2700-3200 mg
  - Phosphorus: ~800-1000 mg

Sunday

- Breakfast:
  Whole-wheat pancakes (2 small, made with ½ cup low-fat milk) topped with sliced banana (½) and a drizzle of maple syrup (1 tbsp).
- Lunch:
  Leftover Homemade Chicken and Vegetable Skewers (same as Saturday dinner).
- Dinner:
  Slow Cooker Pulled Chicken (4 oz) served with mashed sweet potatoes (1 cup) and steamed green beans (1 cup).
- Snacks:
  Plain low-fat yogurt (½ cup), a small handful of blueberries (½ cup).
- Estimated Daily Macros:
  - Calories: ~1500-1700 kcal
  - Carbohydrates: ~180-220 g
  - Proteins: ~90-110 g
  - Fats: ~40-60 g
  - Sodium: ~500-700 mg
  - Potassium: ~2900-3400 mg
  - Phosphorus: ~850-1050 mg

Remember, this is just a starting point. Feel free to swap meals, adjust portion sizes, and incorporate your favorite GERD-friendly recipes. The key is to find a meal planning routine that works for you and helps you enjoy delicious, symptom-free eating while meeting your individual nutritional needs.

Chapter 7: Cooking Tips and Techniques: Flavor Without the Flare-Up

Managing GERD doesn't mean resigning yourself to bland and boring meals. In fact, with a few clever cooking tips and techniques, you can create flavorful and satisfying dishes that are gentle on your stomach and won't trigger those unwelcome symptoms. This chapter will explore strategies for enhancing taste without relying on common irritants, highlight cooking methods that are kind to your digestive system, and offer time-saving techniques for those busy days.

Flavor Enhancement Without Triggering Symptoms: The Art of Subtle Seasoning

One of the biggest concerns for those on a GERD diet is how to make food taste good without using common triggers like spicy peppers, excessive garlic and onions, or acidic tomatoes. The good news is that there's a whole world of flavor you can explore!

- Embrace Fresh Herbs: Fresh herbs like basil, oregano, thyme, rosemary, parsley, cilantro, and dill can add vibrant flavor and aroma to your dishes without the acidity or heat of many spices. Experiment with adding them towards the end of cooking to preserve their freshness.

- Explore Aromatic Vegetables (in moderation): While raw garlic and onions can be triggers for some, cooking them gently can mellow their intensity. Sautéing them in a little olive oil until translucent can provide a subtle savory base for many dishes. Observe your own tolerance.
- Use Mild Spices: Instead of fiery chili powder or cayenne pepper, opt for milder spices like paprika (not smoked), turmeric, cumin (in small amounts for some), ginger, and cinnamon. These can add depth and warmth without the burn.
- Citrus Zest, Not Juice: The zest of lemons, limes, and oranges contains their aromatic oils without the high acidity of the juice. A little zest can brighten up both savory and sweet dishes.
- Vinegar Alternatives: If vinegar is a trigger, try using small amounts of lemon or lime juice (if tolerated) or consider non-acidic alternatives like rice vinegar or a splash of a flavorful broth for deglazing pans.
- Infused Oils: Create your own infused oils by steeping herbs like rosemary or thyme in olive oil. This adds a subtle flavor to your cooking.
- Flavorful Broths and Stocks: Using good quality, low-sodium broths and stocks as a base for soups, stews, and sauces can add significant depth of flavor.
- Umami-Rich Ingredients: Ingredients like mushrooms, soy sauce (in moderation, if tolerated), and nutritional yeast can add a savory "umami" flavor that enhances the overall taste of your meals.

- Sweetness with Caution: If you need a touch of sweetness, opt for small amounts of natural sweeteners like honey or maple syrup, rather than relying heavily on processed sugars.

Cooking Methods That Are Gentle on the Stomach: Kindness in the Kitchen

The way you cook your food can also impact how well it's tolerated by your digestive system. Opting for gentler cooking methods can help reduce fat content and make foods easier to digest.

- Baking: Baking is a great way to cook meats, poultry, fish, and vegetables without adding extra fat. It also helps to retain the natural flavors of the ingredients.
- Broiling and Grilling: These methods use direct heat to cook food quickly and can help render out excess fat. Be mindful of charring, as it can sometimes be irritating.
- Steaming: Steaming is a very gentle cooking method that preserves the nutrients and natural flavors of vegetables, fish, and poultry without the need for added fats.
- Poaching: Poaching involves cooking food gently in a liquid (like water or broth) at a low temperature. This is ideal for delicate proteins like fish and eggs.
- Slow Cooking: Slow cookers are fantastic for making tender and flavorful meals with minimal effort. The long, slow cooking process can break down tougher cuts of meat and meld flavors beautifully. Remember to skim off any excess fat.
- Sautéing with Minimal Oil: When sautéing, use a small amount of olive oil or another healthy fat. Avoid deep-frying altogether.

- Pureeing and Blending: For soups and sauces, blending can create a smoother texture that may be easier to digest for some individuals.

Quick Cooking Techniques for Busy Lives: Flavor in a Flash

Life gets hectic, but that doesn't mean you have to compromise on your GERD-friendly diet. Here are some quick cooking techniques to get healthy and flavorful meals on the table in a flash:

- Stir-Frying: Using a wok or large skillet, stir-frying lean proteins and non-acidic vegetables in a small amount of oil is a quick and versatile way to create a meal. Prepare your ingredients (chop vegetables, slice protein) ahead of time for even faster cooking.
- Sheet Pan Meals: Toss vegetables and lean protein with a little olive oil and herbs, then roast them all together on a single sheet pan for easy cleanup.
- One-Pot Wonders: Soups, stews, and pasta dishes cooked in a single pot minimize cleanup and are often quick to assemble.
- Microwave Magic (Use Wisely): While not ideal for all foods, the microwave can be a useful tool for reheating leftovers or quickly steaming vegetables.
- Pre-Cooked Proteins: Keep pre-cooked chicken breasts, canned tuna or salmon, or hard-boiled eggs on hand for quick additions to salads or wraps.
- Frozen Vegetables: Frozen vegetables are just as nutritious as fresh and can be cooked quickly by steaming, microwaving, or adding directly to stir-fries or soups.
- Quick Grain Options: Cook quinoa, couscous, or microwaveable rice for fast and easy carbohydrate sources.
- Salad Assembly: Combine pre-washed greens with your choice of lean protein, non-acidic vegetables, and a light, GERD-friendly dressing for a quick and refreshing meal.

By mastering these flavor-enhancing strategies, gentle cooking methods, and quick techniques, you can create a repertoire of delicious and satisfying GERD-friendly meals that fit your lifestyle and keep your symptoms at bay. Cooking with GERD in mind doesn't have to be a limitation; it can be an opportunity to explore new flavors and healthier ways of preparing your favorite foods.

Chapter 8: Coping with Dietary Restrictions: Thriving in a Food-Focused World

Living with GERD often means navigating dietary restrictions that can sometimes feel isolating or challenging, especially in social situations or when cooking for family members with different needs. However, with thoughtful strategies and open communication, you can successfully manage your diet while still enjoying social connections and creating harmonious mealtimes at home. This chapter offers practical advice on coping with these dietary adjustments and thriving within them.

Navigating Social Situations with GERD: Enjoying Life Beyond Your Kitchen

Social events often revolve around food, which can create anxiety for individuals managing GERD. Here are some tips to navigate these situations with confidence and comfort:

- Plan Ahead Whenever Possible: If you know you'll be attending a party or restaurant, try to find out what kind of food will be served. Many restaurants have their menus online. This allows you to identify potential GERD-friendly options in advance.
- Communicate Your Needs Discreetly: Don't hesitate to politely inform the host or server about your dietary restrictions. You don't need to go into extensive detail, but a simple "I have a medical condition that requires me to avoid certain foods like [mention a key trigger or two]" can be helpful. Most people are understanding and willing to accommodate.
- Offer to Bring a Dish: If you're attending a potluck, offering to bring a GERD-friendly dish ensures you'll have at least one safe and delicious option to enjoy. This can also be a great way to introduce others to flavorful alternatives.
- Focus on Socializing, Not Just the Food: Remember that the primary purpose of social gatherings is connection and enjoyment. Shift your focus to conversations, activities, and the company of others, rather than solely on what you can or cannot eat.
- Make Smart Choices: When faced with a buffet or a variety of dishes, carefully scan the options and choose items that are likely to be safe. Look for lean proteins, steamed or baked vegetables, and simple preparations. Avoid fried foods, creamy sauces, and anything that looks overly spicy or acidic.
- Don't Be Afraid to Ask Questions: If you're unsure about an ingredient or preparation method, don't hesitate to politely ask the host or server for clarification. It's better to be informed than to risk triggering your symptoms.

- Carry Safe Snacks: If you're concerned about limited options, discreetly carry a few GERD-friendly snacks like plain crackers, a banana, or a small bag of nuts to tide you over.
- BYOB (Bring Your Own Beverage): If certain beverages are triggers (like alcohol or carbonated drinks), consider bringing your own safe alternative, like plain water or herbal tea in a thermos.
- Practice Mindful Eating: Even when safe options are available, eat slowly and pay attention to your body's signals. Overeating can trigger reflux, regardless of the food.
- Be Kind to Yourself: It's okay if you can't always adhere perfectly to your diet in social situations. Do your best, enjoy the event, and get back on track with your regular eating plan afterward.

Involving Family in Meal Preparation: A Team Effort for Digestive Health

When you live with others, involving your family in meal preparation can foster understanding, support, and make it easier to maintain your GERD diet.

- Educate Your Family: Explain to your family members why certain foods trigger your symptoms and the importance of following a GERD-friendly diet for your health and well-being. The more they understand, the more supportive they are likely to be.
- Plan Meals Together: Involve your family in the meal planning process. Ask for their input on GERD-friendly recipes they might enjoy. This can make them feel included and more invested in the meals you prepare.

- Assign Age-Appropriate Tasks: Even younger children can help with tasks like washing vegetables, setting the table, or stirring ingredients. This not only lightens your load but also educates them about healthy eating.
- Cook Together: Make meal preparation a family activity. This can be a fun way to spend time together and ensures that everyone is aware of the ingredients and cooking methods being used.
- Focus on Shared Meals: Aim to create meals that everyone can enjoy, with minor modifications if necessary. For example, you might prepare a baked chicken dish with roasted vegetables that is suitable for everyone.
- Be Open to Compromise: While your health needs are paramount, be open to occasional compromises when possible. Perhaps a family favorite that is usually a trigger can be made with modifications or enjoyed in a very small portion on a special occasion.
- Express Gratitude for Support: Acknowledge and appreciate your family's efforts to support your dietary needs. Positive reinforcement can go a long way in maintaining a supportive environment.

Cooking for Mixed Dietary Needs: Balancing GERD with Other Preferences

Many households have members with varying dietary needs and preferences. Cooking for mixed needs can seem challenging, but with a few strategic approaches, you can create meals that cater to everyone.

- Identify Common Ground: Focus on meals that naturally align with a GERD-friendly diet and other dietary needs.

Lean proteins, non-acidic vegetables, and whole grains can often form the base of many dishes.

- Utilize Adaptable Components: Prepare main components of a meal in a GERD-friendly way and then offer optional additions or sauces on the side for those with different preferences. For example, you could serve plain grilled chicken with a side of spicy salsa for those who can tolerate it.
- "Deconstruct" Meals: For dishes like tacos or salads, lay out the individual components separately, allowing each person to build their own meal according to their dietary needs and preferences.
- Prepare Separate Sides: If a particular side dish is a trigger for you but enjoyed by others, consider preparing a small, separate portion for them while you enjoy a GERD-friendly alternative.
- Modify Recipes Strategically: Look for ways to adapt family favorite recipes to be more GERD-friendly. This might involve using less fat, substituting acidic ingredients, or omitting common triggers.
- Embrace One-Pot or Sheet Pan Meals with Variations: You can often divide a sheet pan or pot and season different sections according to individual preferences.
- Plan "Theme Nights": Consider having theme nights (like "Build-Your-Own Salad Night" or "Grain Bowl Night") where everyone can customize their meal with a variety of safe and enjoyable ingredients.
- Don't Be Afraid of Leftovers: Cooking larger, adaptable meals can lead to leftovers that can be customized for different dietary needs for lunch the next day.

Coping with dietary restrictions due to GERD is a journey that requires patience, communication, and a willingness to adapt. By employing these strategies, you can navigate social situations with greater ease, involve your family in your dietary journey, and successfully cook for mixed dietary needs, ensuring that mealtimes remain a positive and inclusive experience for everyone.

Chapter 9: Additional Resources: Your Continued Journey to Wellness

Congratulations on taking proactive steps towards managing your GERD through dietary changes! The information in this book provides a solid foundation, but the journey to understanding and living well with GERD is ongoing. This chapter offers a curated list of additional resources to support you further, providing access to more recipes, up-to-date information, and valuable community connections.

Recommended GERD Health and Nutrition Websites: Reliable Information at Your Fingertips

The internet can be a wealth of information, but it's crucial to rely on credible sources, especially when it comes to your health. Here are some reputable websites that offer valuable information on GERD, nutrition, and digestive health:

- National Institute of Diabetes and Digestive and Kidney Diseases (NIDDK) (https://www.niddk.nih.gov/): A leading government agency providing comprehensive information on GERD, its causes, symptoms, treatment, and related research.

- American College of Gastroenterology (ACG) (https://gi.org/): The professional organization for gastroenterologists, offering clinical guidelines, patient education resources, and the latest advancements in digestive health.
- Mayo Clinic (https://www.mayoclinic.org/): A trusted medical center providing detailed information on various health conditions, including GERD, with practical advice on lifestyle modifications and dietary management.
- World Gastroenterology Organisation (WGO) (https://www.worldgastroenterology.org/): A global organization offering guidelines and resources on digestive health, including GERD, from an international perspective.
- Academy of Nutrition and Dietetics (https://www.eatright.org/): The professional organization for registered dietitians and nutrition experts, offering evidence-based information on healthy eating and managing various health conditions through diet. Search their site for articles and resources on GERD.

Support Groups and Community Resources: Connecting with Others on the Journey

Living with a chronic condition like GERD can sometimes feel isolating. Connecting with others who understand your experiences can provide invaluable emotional support, practical tips, and a sense of community. Here are some ways to find support:

- Online GERD Support Groups: Numerous online forums and social media groups are dedicated to individuals living with GERD. These platforms offer a space to share experiences, ask questions, and connect with others facing similar challenges. Search for "GERD support group" on platforms like Facebook or Reddit. (Always exercise caution and consult your healthcare provider for medical advice shared in online forums.)

- Local Support Groups: Check with your healthcare provider or local hospitals and clinics to see if there are any in-person GERD support groups in your area. Meeting face-to-face can provide a strong sense of community.
- Patient Advocacy Organizations: Organizations focused on digestive health often have resources and may be able to connect you with support networks. Search for national or regional digestive disease advocacy groups.
- Registered Dietitian or Nutritionist: Working with a registered dietitian who specializes in gastrointestinal disorders can provide personalized guidance and support[1] in navigating your GERD diet and addressing any nutritional concerns.
- Therapist or Counselor: Dealing with a chronic condition can be emotionally challenging. A therapist or counselor can provide support and coping strategies to manage any stress or anxiety related to your GERD and dietary restrictions.

Remember, you are not alone in managing GERD. By utilizing these additional resources, you can continue to expand your knowledge, discover new ways to enjoy delicious food, and connect with a supportive community that understands your journey. Embrace these tools as you continue on your path to heartburn-free living and enhanced wellness.

Conclusion: Embracing a Flavorful, Heartburn-Free Future

Congratulations! You've reached the end of *GERD Diet Essentials*, and in doing so, you've armed yourself with a wealth of knowledge and practical strategies to navigate the world of GERD and nutrition. This journey of understanding your body and making informed food choices is a powerful one, and you should be proud of the steps you've taken.

Empowering Your Journey to Manage GERD: Taking Control of Your Well-being

Our aim throughout this book has been to empower you – to provide you with the clarity, confidence, and tools you need to take control of your GERD symptoms and live a life where delicious food and comfort can coexist. We've explored the fundamentals of GERD, delved into the specifics of a GERD-friendly diet, offered practical meal planning and cooking tips, and provided guidance on navigating the social and familial aspects of dietary restrictions.

Remember that managing GERD is not about rigid rules and deprivation. It's about becoming more attuned to your body's unique responses, making mindful choices, and discovering a sustainable way of eating that nourishes you without triggering discomfort. The food lists and recipes provided are a starting point, a foundation upon which you can build a personalized and enjoyable eating plan.

The journey may have its ups and downs. You might encounter new trigger foods or have days when symptoms flare up despite your best efforts. This is a normal part of managing a chronic condition. The key is to remain patient with yourself, learn from these experiences, and continue to apply the principles and strategies you've learned. Don't be discouraged by setbacks; view them as opportunities to further refine your understanding of your own body's needs.

We encourage you to continue exploring the resources provided in the previous chapter. The online world offers a wealth of recipes, support communities, and up-to-date information that can further enhance your journey. Connecting with others who understand what you're going through can be incredibly valuable, and staying informed about the latest research can empower you to make the best decisions for your health.

Thank You and Encouragement for Healthy Living: A Toast to Your Well-being

From my heart, thank you for allowing me, Catherine Rosales-Holt, to be your guide on this important journey. As a registered nurse specializing in gastroenterology, my greatest hope is to see you thrive – to enjoy meals without fear, to feel comfortable and energized, and to live a full and vibrant life.

Remember that you are not defined by your GERD. It is a condition you manage, and with the right knowledge and tools, you can live well despite it. Embrace the principles of mindful eating, gentle cooking, and proactive planning. Celebrate the small victories, and be kind to yourself along the way.

I sincerely hope that *GERD Diet Essentials* has provided you with the practical support and encouragement you need to embark on a path towards a healthier, happier, and more heartburn-free future. Here's to delicious meals, comfortable days, and a continued journey of well-being. You've got this!

Thank You For Reading!

I sincerely appreciate you investing your time and energy in *GERD Diet Essentials*. My goal in writing this book was to provide you with practical and supportive guidance for navigating the GERD diet.

If you found this book beneficial and feel it could help others, I would be deeply grateful if you would consider leaving a review on Amazon. Your feedback is invaluable and helps spread the word to those who may also be seeking relief.

Leaving a review is easy! Simply visit:

https://go.binnovatedigital.com/GERDFoodlist

Or Scan the QR code below to go directly to the review page:

Your support means the world to me. Thank you very much!

Love,

-Catherine

Reference

- National Institute of Diabetes and Digestive and Kidney Diseases (NIDDK): Provides comprehensive information on GERD, its causes, symptoms, and management.[1] (https://www.niddk.nih.gov/)
- American College of Gastroenterology (ACG): Offers clinical guidelines and patient education resources on GERD.[2] (https://gi.org/)
- National Institute of Diabetes and Digestive and Kidney Diseases (NIDDK): "GER & GERD." (https://www.niddk.nih.gov/health-information/digestive-diseases/acid-reflux-ger-gerd)
- American College of Gastroenterology (ACG): "GERD: A Patient's Guide." (https://gi.org/topics/acid-reflux-gerd/)
- Mayo Clinic: "GERD (gastroesophageal reflux disease) - Symptoms and causes." (https://www.mayoclinic.org/diseases-conditions/gerd/symptoms-causes/syc-20361901)
- World Gastroenterology Organisation (WGO): "GERD Global Guidelines." (https://www.worldgastroenterology.org/guidelines/gerd)
- Johns Hopkins Medicine: "GERD Diet: Foods That Help with Acid Reflux (Heartburn)." (https://www.hopkinsmedicine.org/health/wellness-and-prevention/gerd-diet-foods-that-help-with-acid-reflux-heartburn)
- Mayo Clinic: "Acid reflux (GERD) - Lifestyle and home remedies." (https://www.mayoclinic.org/diseases-conditions/gerd/diagnosis-treatment/drc-20361905)

- National Institute of Diabetes and Digestive and Kidney Diseases (NIDDK): "Eating, Diet, & Nutrition for GER & GERD." (https://www.niddk.nih.gov/health-information/digestive-diseases/acid-reflux-ger-gerd/eating-diet-nutrition)
- Academy of Nutrition and Dietetics: Provides resources and information on meal planning and healthy eating. (https://www.eatright.org/)
- Mayo Clinic: Offers practical tips for healthy meal planning. (https://www.mayoclinic.org/healthy-lifestyle/nutrition-and-healthy-eating/in-depth/meal-planning/art-20048172)
- Various Health and Nutrition Websites: Many reputable websites offer guides and tips on meal prepping and healthy eating. Search for "healthy meal planning tips" and "GERD-friendly recipes" for more inspiration.
- Academy of Nutrition and Dietetics: Provides resources and information on meal planning and healthy eating. (https://www.eatright.org/)
- Mayo Clinic: Offers practical tips for healthy meal planning. (https://www.mayoclinic.org/healthy-lifestyle/nutrition-and-healthy-eating/in-depth/meal-planning/art-20048172)
- USDA FoodData Central: A comprehensive source for nutrient information on various foods. (https://fdc.nal.usda.gov/) *Note: Individual food nutrient values were estimated using this database for the sample meal plan.*
- Various Health and Nutrition Websites: Many reputable websites offer guides and tips on meal prepping and healthy eating. Search for "healthy meal planning tips" and "GERD-friendly recipes" for more inspiration.
- Cleveland Clinic: "Acid Reflux Diet: What to Eat (and Avoid)." (https://my.clevelandclinic.org/health/diseases/17019-acid-reflux-gerd-diet)

- Healthline: "The GERD Diet: Foods to Eat and Avoid." (https://www.healthline.com/health/gerd/diet)
- Various Culinary Resources: Websites and cookbooks focusing on healthy cooking techniques and flavor development using herbs and spices.

1. How Dietary Fat Affects GERD Symptoms:

- Mechanism: Health resources like Cooper University Health Care, GERDHelp.com, Cleveland Clinic, and the American Society for Gastrointestinal Endoscopy (ASGE) explain that high-fat foods can trigger GERD symptoms in two main ways:
    - They can relax the lower esophageal sphincter (LES), the valve that normally keeps stomach contents from backing up into the esophagus.
    - They slow down stomach emptying, meaning food and acid stay in the stomach longer, increasing the opportunity for reflux to occur.
- Increased Risk: Fatty meals, especially large ones, are frequently linked to worsening GERD symptoms (Cleveland Clinic, Healthline).
- Reduce Overall Fat: Many sources recommend decreasing total dietary fat intake to help prevent reflux (Healthline, Patient.gastro.org). This includes limiting saturated fats (often found in meat and dairy) and avoiding trans fats (found in processed foods, margarines) (Medical News Today, Patient.gastro.org).
- Choose Lean Proteins: Opt for lean meats like skinless chicken and turkey, fish, beans, lentils, and tofu. Preparation methods like baking, grilling, broiling, or poaching are preferred over frying (Medical News Today, Healthline, Mount Elizabeth Hospitals, AboutGERD.org/IFFGD).

- Select Lower-Fat Dairy: Choose low-fat or nonfat milk, yogurt, and cheese, or plant-based alternatives (Verywell Health, Baptist Health, Healthline). Egg whites are often better tolerated than higher-fat egg yolks (Medical News Today, AboutGERD.org/IFFGD).
- Include Healthy Fats (in Moderation): Unsaturated fats found in avocados, nuts, seeds, olive oil, and fatty fish are generally better choices than saturated or trans fats. However, even these should be consumed in moderation as all fats are calorie-dense and large amounts might still trigger symptoms for some (Medical News Today, Patient.gastro.org, GERDHelp.com).

3. High-Fat Foods Often Recommended to Limit or Avoid:

- Based on multiple sources (including Cooper Health, GERDHelp.com, Healthline, Medical News Today, Michigan Medicine, Mount Elizabeth Hospitals, ASGE), common high-fat trigger foods include:
    - Fried foods (French fries, onion rings, fried chicken)
    - Fatty cuts of meat (red meat like beef, pork, lamb, bacon, sausage)
    - Full-fat dairy products (whole milk, butter, regular cheese, cream, sour cream, rich ice cream)
    - Creamy sauces, gravies, and dressings
    - Pastries, doughnuts, chocolate, cookies, cakes, potato chips
    - Fast food items

4. Reading Nutrition Labels:

- Check Serving Size: It's crucial to note the serving size and servings per container, as all other values are based on this amount. Eating multiple servings increases your intake of fat, calories, etc. (GERDHelp.com - Senior Nutrition Guide, Pritikin).

- Compare Fat Content: While a specific "grams of fat" cut-off isn't universally recommended for all GERD patients per item, reading labels helps you compare similar products. Choose options lower in "Total Fat" and "Saturated Fat" (advice synthesized from general low-fat recommendations).
- Look at Ingredients: Identify hidden fats (like lard, butter, shortening, certain oils) and other potential triggers like chocolate, peppermint, caffeine, high amounts of citric acid, tomato products, onion, or garlic powder (Cooper Health, ASGE, Pritikin).
- Consider Fat Percentage/Calories: Some sources suggest being mindful of foods where fat contributes a large percentage of the total calories (Pritikin suggests a calculation or rule of thumb for their program: ≤2g fat per 100 calories). Patient.gastro.org recommends limiting saturated fat to less than 7% of total daily calories.

5. Individual Tolerance and Meal Context:

- Triggers Vary: Experts emphasize that trigger foods are highly individual. What causes reflux in one person may not affect another (Healthline, Michigan Medicine, Patient.gastro.org, Mount Elizabeth Hospitals).
- Food Diary: Keeping a detailed food diary (noting foods eaten, amounts, timing, and symptoms) is frequently recommended to identify personal triggers and tolerance levels (Healthline, Michigan Medicine, Pepcid).
- Overall Meal Matters: The total amount of fat in an entire meal is often more significant than the fat content of a single component (general principle derived from advice to avoid large, high-fat meals).

6. Importance of Meal Size and Timing:

- Smaller, Frequent Meals: Eating smaller meals more frequently throughout the day, rather than two or three large meals, is consistently advised to reduce pressure on the stomach and LES (Healthline, Michigan Medicine, Pepcid, Patient.gastro.org).

- Avoid Eating Before Bed: Allow 2-3 hours between your last meal or snack and lying down to give your stomach time to empty (Healthline, Michigan Medicine, Vinmec).

Made in United States
Troutdale, OR
11/03/2026

56847554R00116